Live Longer, Feel Younger

1,001 Ways to Keep Your Belly Lean, Memory Sharp, Senses Keen, and Heart Healthy Into Your 90s and Beyond

Publisher's Note

The editors of FC&A have taken careful measures to ensure the accuracy and usefulness of the information in this book. While every attempt was made to assure accuracy, some Web sites, addresses, telephone numbers, and other information may have changed since printing.

This book is intended for general information only. It does not constitute medical advice or practice. We cannot guarantee the safety or effectiveness of any treatment or advice mentioned. Readers are urged to consult with their health care professionals and get their approval before undertaking therapies suggested by information in this book, keeping in mind that errors in the text may occur as in all publications and that new findings may supercede older information.

> *"Finally, be strong in the Lord and in the strength of His might."*
>
> *Ephesians 6:10*

FC&A Medical Publishing®
103 Clover Green
Peachtree City, GA 30269

Produced by the staff of FC&A

ISBN 978-1-932470-97-0

Table of contents

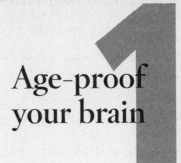

Age-proof your brain

Hot drinks that help your brain

Whether you jump-start your day with a piping hot mug of coffee or relax in the afternoon with a soothing cup of tea, you're doing your brain a favor. Several studies suggest that drinking coffee or tea can protect you from Alzheimer's disease and mental decline.

Coffee perks up your brain. You've heard of a midlife crisis. But drinking coffee during middle age may help you avoid a brain crisis later. In a study of 1,409 people, Finnish researchers found that those who drank moderate amounts of coffee around age 50 were much less likely to develop Alzheimer's disease or other types of dementia later in life.

Moderate coffee drinkers — those who drank three to five cups a day — had the lowest risk. They slashed their risk of dementia by 65 to 70 percent and their risk of Alzheimer's by 62 to 64 percent compared to low coffee drinkers, or those who drank zero to two cups a day. A French study found similar results. Women who drank more than three cups of coffee a day had less decline in verbal recall and memory than those who drank a cup a day or less.

While researchers aren't sure why coffee helps, they suspect it could have something to do with coffee's antioxidants. A recent University of North Dakota study of rabbits shed more light on how coffee may work. Alzheimer's disease may be caused or aggravated by a breakdown in the blood-brain barrier, a filter that protects the brain from potentially harmful substances in the bloodstream while letting in oxygen and other essential nutrients. High levels of cholesterol in the blood can make this barrier leaky.

The 12-week study, which involved feeding rabbits a high-cholesterol diet, found that caffeine helped protect against disruptions to the blood-brain barrier. The caffeine dosage used in the study — 3 milligrams — is equivalent to one cup of coffee a day for an average-size person. Researchers say just one cup of coffee a day might be enough to help prevent Alzheimer's.

Tea time slows mental decline. For a sharper mind — no matter what your age — make sure you sip two cups of green tea daily. In a Japanese study of 1,000 people age 70 or older, those who drank at least two cups of green tea daily had the lowest risk of mental impairment, as measured by tests of mental status. In fact, they were 54 percent less likely to show signs of impairment than those who drank three cups of green tea or less a week. An antioxidant in green tea called epigallocatechin-3-gallate, or EGCG, may deserve the credit. Lab and animal studies show it can help prevent the formation of plaques associated with Alzheimer's disease and Parkinson's disease.

But it's not just green tea that seems to give your brain a boost. A study of older Chinese people found that regular tea consumption, especially of black or oolong tea, was associated with less risk of mental impairment or decline. Oolong and green tea also helped reverse mental impairment and lessen brain degeneration in mice, probably because of strong antioxidant activity. Theanine, an amino acid found almost exclusively in tea, helps people focus and perform better on tests. When combined with caffeine, it works even better. That could help explain some of tea's brain-boosting powers.

Before you take a sip. Coffee and tea are safe for most people, but not for everyone. Don't combine caffeinated drinks with monoamine oxidase inhibitors, an older class of antidepressants. It may trigger a spike in blood pressure. You may also want to limit caffeine if you have heart disease, osteoporosis, anxiety, heartburn, gastritis, or headaches.

Keep your brain young with juice

You don't have to lose your memories. Just remember to eat plenty of fruits and vegetables. Packed with antioxidants that fight aging, nature's sweet treats do wonders for your brain. Whole fruits like apples, bananas, oranges, plums, grapes, and cherries offer plenty of antioxidant protection against oxidative stress that can lead to nerve degeneration and Alzheimer's disease. But you don't need to bite into a piece of fruit to reap its benefits.

Beverage breakthrough. A recent Vanderbilt study suggests that juice is better than fruits and veggies. If you want to stay healthy and independent into your 90s, this is one study you definitely want to know about. The study followed 1,836 Japanese Americans in Seattle for up to 10 years. Those who drank fruit or vegetable juice at least three times a week had a 76 percent lower risk of developing Alzheimer's than those who drank juice less than once a week.

Polyphenols, antioxidant chemicals found mostly in the skins and peels of fruits and vegetables, probably give juices their power. Some polyphenols can cross the blood-brain barrier, a filter that protects the brain from harmful substances and oxidative damage. Some also have powerful anti-inflammatory properties. Other components of juice, including antioxidant vitamins, folate and minerals, may also help. Whatever the reason for juice's benefit, you can slash your risk of Alzheimer's with just three glasses a week.

Another study, which measured the phenolic content of several commercially available fruit juices and drinks, found that purple grape juice had the highest concentration of polyphenols — about the same as a light red wine. It also had the highest antioxidant capacity. Other good choices included cranberry juice, grapefruit juice, and cloudy apple juice.

Apple juice also showed promise in lab tests on mice. In a recent study, mice who received the human equivalent of two glasses of apple juice a day for a month produced less beta-amyloid, a protein fragment that forms plaques in the brains of people with Alzheimer's disease. Apple juice and grape juice — great choices to help you preserve your memory.

'Berry' good news. Worried about your memory? Blueberries can keep it sharp. That's because they're loaded with polyphenols, especially anthocyanins, which give blueberries their color.

In Tufts University studies, rats given blueberry or strawberry extracts performed better on maze tests that measure memory and learning. Polyphenols from berries accumulate in the brain after long-term consumption. They also interact with aging brain cells to help them maintain proper functioning.

One compound found in berries and grapes called pterostilbene prevented oxidative stress in lab tests and reversed mental decline and improved working memory in aging rats. British researchers found similar encouraging results with blueberries.

Scale back aging with fish

Fishing for an easy way to stay young? Look no further than your local fish market. Omega-3 fatty acids found in fish can help defend against mental decline, Alzheimer's, Parkinson's disease, and depression.

Gills save skills. Several studies suggest that eating fish can help preserve your mental skills. A Norwegian study found that older people who ate just 10 grams, which is about a third of an ounce, of fish or more a day did much better on mental tests than those who ate less. For best results, aim for 75 grams, or about 3 ounces, of fish each day.

Dutch researchers reported a link between higher blood levels of omega-3 and lower mental decline. Older people who had the highest levels of omega-3 in their blood at the start of the study demonstrated less mental decline over the next three years, particularly in tests that involved thinking speed.

It's not just how much fish you eat that matters. How you prepare it also makes a difference. Broiled or baked tuna and other types of fish high in omega-3 fatty acids may help lower the risk of mental decline in older adults. In one study, people who ate this type of fish three or more times a week slashed their risk of having small brain lesions that can cause loss of thinking skills, stroke, or dementia by 26 percent. But fried fish had no impact.

Mackerel helps your mood. As a population's omega-3 consumption decreases, its incidence of depression increases. There are a few possible explanations for this. Scientists suspect that your brain converts eicosapentaenoic acid (EPA), an omega-3 fatty acid, into chemicals your brain needs, such as prostaglandins or leukotrienes. Or maybe omega-3 fatty acids affect the signaling in your brain cells by activating or blocking certain receptors. Taking supplements that contain 1.5 to 2 grams of EPA a day has been shown to elevate the mood of depressed people, but more than 3 grams doesn't increase the benefit.

One recent study found that eating fish may help women lower their risk for chronic depressive symptoms. Those who ate the most fish reduced their risk by 25 percent compared to those who ate the least. Another study found that supplemental EPA eased psychological distress and depressive symptoms in menopausal women. As a bonus, it also helped reduce hot flashes. On the other hand, a French study reported that eating fatty fish may lower the risk of depression for men and nonsmokers — but not for people who smoke.

Why does fish benefit your brain? About two-thirds of your brain tissue is composed of fats, so it's important to get the right kinds. Healthy fats, like the omega-3 fatty acids found in fish, promote communication among brain cells and keep cell membranes elastic. An omega-3 fatty acid called docosahexaenoic acid (DHA) provides fluidity, or the ability to transport signals within the brain. It also helps synapses — the junctions between nerve cells — change, which is the basis for memory. Diets rich in DHA have also been shown to protect against Alzheimer's, Parkinson's disease, and depression.

Good sources of omega-3 fatty acids include anchovies, herring, lake trout, mackerel, salmon, sardines, and tuna. Make an effort to eat fish two or three times a week, and you'll feed your brain as well as your belly. You can also get some omega-3 from nuts and dark leafy greens.

Solution for landlubbers. Of course, not everyone likes the taste of fish. Luckily, even landlubbers can benefit from omega-3 fatty acids by taking fish oil supplements. In fact, one small study found that 1 gram of EPA together with the prescription antidepressant Prozac works better for depression than either remedy by itself.

Unlike with fish, you don't have to worry about high levels of mercury, lead, or other contaminants with supplements. But you should be careful if you take blood-thinning or blood pressure-lowering drugs, since fish oil will enhance those effects.

Another reason to avoid a high-fat diet

Your brain needs some fat, but make sure it's the right kind. A Canadian study of mice studied the effects of a diet with a low ratio of omega-3 to omega-6 fatty acids. Mice were fed either a low-fat or high-fat diet. Researchers found that a high-fat diet, along with a low omega-6 to omega-3 ratio, promoted changes in the brain like those found in Alzheimer's disease.

To improve your fat ratio, eat more fish, especially fatty fish like salmon, mackerel, herring, and tuna. You should also avoid deep-fried foods, margarine, and salad dressings that contain corn oil or soybean oil. Use olive or canola oil instead.

Heart-healthy diet staves off dementia

Fruits, vegetables, and fish provide plenty of brain benefits on their own, but they're even more powerful when you make them part of a healthy diet. Omega-3 fatty acids from fish and antioxidants from fruits and vegetables are possibly the two most powerful, and most overlooked, all-natural anti-aging agents in the world. Discover them both in the Mediterranean diet.

In addition to plenty of fruits, veggies, and fish, the Mediterranean diet emphasizes nuts, grains, seeds, beans, olive oil, and moderate wine consumption, which means a glass of wine a day for women and up to two glasses a day for men. It also features very little meat and dairy products. It all adds up to a recipe for a healthier heart — and a sharper mind.

A recent study found that people who followed a Mediterranean diet and exercised had a 60 percent lower risk of developing Alzheimer's disease compared to those who did neither. An earlier study by the same researchers found that sticking to a Mediterranean diet lowered both the risk of developing mild mental impairment and the risk of mild mental impairment progressing to Alzheimer's.

A word of caution — if you don't drink alcohol, don't start. Alcohol raises your risk for breast cancer, cirrhosis of the liver, and other serious health problems. Instead, add more grapes and grape juice to your day.

4 flavorful ways to protect your brain

Herbs and spices add flavor to any meal. But they also spice up your defenses against Alzheimer's disease and depression. Here are a few tasty ways to protect your brain.

Sample some sage. A new study reveals that this little-known herbal medication can help reduce dementia symptoms. It makes people more cheerful, too. In the study, sage extract helped people with mild to moderate Alzheimer's disease. The equivalent of about 1.5 teaspoons of sage a day led to significant improvements in thought processes after 16 weeks of treatment. Sage works by boosting levels of acetylcholine, a chemical produced by the brain that is essential for short-term memory function. Even if you don't have memory problems, sage can help by improving your mood.

Try turmeric. This spice gives curry dishes their distinctive yellow color. It may also prevent and control Alzheimer's disease by reducing the buildup of harmful proteins in the brain. About 4 teaspoons a day should do the trick.

Grab some garlic. Lab tests show garlic extract prevents amyloid beta deposits in the brain, a key feature of Alzheimer's disease.

While both fresh and boiled garlic stopped amyloid plaques from forming, only the fresh garlic broke up already existing deposits. Garlic's powerful sulfur compounds, along with its antioxidant properties, likely team up to protect your brain. Just eating more garlic may help prevent or delay Alzheimer's.

Search for saffron. This costly spice, which gives paella, a popular rice dish in Spain, its yellow color, may be worth the hefty price. Studies show both the petal and stamen of saffron have powerful antidepressant effects. In fact, 30 milligrams of saffron may be just as effective as Prozac and other common antidepressants for treating mild to moderate depression.

Fill up on folate to fight dementia

Want a sharp brain at 70? It may be as simple as eating more spinach and asparagus. That's because these two vegetables are packed with folate, the heart-saving, brain-boosting, stroke-stopping, mood-enhancing vitamin that you absolutely shouldn't miss out on.

In a recent Korean study, older people with a folate deficiency had more than triple the risk of dementia. Even those with lower folate levels that didn't quite qualify as deficient were at higher risk. Researchers noted that weight loss, which often occurs early in dementia, may be partially responsible for changes in folate levels. In addition, a Dutch study found that higher blood levels of folate led to better performance on mental tests.

But it's not quite that simple. Folate is closely related to homocysteine, a by-product of protein metabolism. A deficiency of folate can lead to higher levels of homocysteine. High levels of homocysteine have been linked to mental decline, dementia, and depression, as well as heart disease and stroke — the same conditions linked to low levels of folate. So it's hard to say whether low folate levels or high homocysteine levels are to blame. Folate does play a role in essential fatty acid metabolism, which could help explain its effect on brain function.

If you're forgetful, irritable, or you can't sleep, you may have a folate deficiency. Symptoms include depression and mental confusion, along with fatigue, irritability, and headache. Get more folate and you could feel much better in as little as two days.

Here's an easy way to get extra folate into your diet. Toss up a folate-rich salad. It could be one of the most important nutritional decisions you'll ever make. You'll be amazed to find out how many of these ingredients can help prevent the devastating effects of Alzheimer's disease. Choose your favorites. You can't go wrong with any combination of beets, spinach, asparagus, leafy greens, black-eyed peas, lentils, beans, red or green peppers, artichokes, papaya, and seeds. You can also find folate in liver and enriched breads, cereal, pasta, and grains.

Short-circuit memory loss and depression

Folate isn't the only B vitamin that helps your brain. Vitamin B12 and vitamin B3 also play important anti-aging roles. Find out why you need to get more of these key B vitamins.

Maximize your memory. In one recent study, people with low levels of vitamin B12 were six times more likely to show signs of brain atrophy, or shrinkage, which can lead to memory loss or Alzheimer's disease. Another study found that high levels of methylmalonic acid, which rises when B12 levels get too low, predicts a faster decline in mental health.

You can get more vitamin B12 in your diet through meat, fish, fortified cereals, and milk. In fact, drinking just two glasses of milk each day could help guard against Alzheimer's, according to a recent University of Oxford study. Skim milk also does the trick.

Nicotinamide, a form of vitamin B3 or niacin, helped mice with dementia perform memory tasks in a recent study. When the mice were given nicotinamide in their drinking water, they performed the tasks as if they'd never had dementia. This form of B3 also gave mice without dementia a boost in short-term memory. It likely works by lowering levels of a protein that contributes to tangles that can clog brain cells and lead to Alzheimer's. Aim for 14 milligrams (mg) of B3 each day. You can find it in dairy products, poultry, fish, nuts, lean meats, eggs, and whole grains.

Improve your mood. Vitamin B12 may also help with depression. Women with low B12 levels are more than twice as likely to develop depression as those with normal levels, and studies show that people given 0.4 mg a day of B12 exhibit fewer depression symptoms.

In addition to food sources, you can get synthetic B12 from supplements or a multivitamin. As you get older and produce less stomach acid, you may have trouble absorbing B12 from foods. Just don't fall for gimmicky vitamin drinks, which provide very little nutrition. You'd have to drink about five cans of vitamin-enriched soda to get all your B vitamins. Some vitamins break down in an acidic environment, like cola, and vitamin waters often come packed with added sugar. It's best to get your B vitamins from a healthy diet.

Defend your brain with vitamin D

The sunshine vitamin really shines when it comes to fighting dementia and depression. Boosting your vitamin D intake may lower your risk for several brain-related conditions.

Dementia. A British study found that low blood levels of vitamin D may boost your risk for dementia. In a study of older people, those with the lowest levels of vitamin D were 2.3 times more likely to have mental impairment compared to those with the highest levels.

In another study, people with high levels of vitamin D performed better on tests of "executive function" — the mental ability involved in planning, organizing, paying attention to details, forming concepts, and thinking abstractly. They were also less likely to have damage to small blood vessels in the brain or disease in the brain's white matter.

While no direct link has been established, receptors for vitamin D have been found in the areas of the brain involved in complex planning, processing, and the formation of new memories.

Parkinson's disease. Emory University researchers discovered that people with Parkinson's disease were more likely to have insufficient levels of vitamin D than healthy people or those with Alzheimer's disease. Because of mobility problems, people with Parkinson's might get less sun exposure, which could explain the deficiency. But low vitamin D levels may also contribute to Parkinson's, and boosting your intake may help.

Depression. Spending more time in the sun may also help lower your risk of depression. Dutch researchers found that older people with depression had lower blood levels of vitamin D. Lower vitamin D levels also meant more severe depression. Of course, depression could lead to low vitamin D status, rather than the other way around. If you're depressed, maybe you're spending less time outdoors or neglecting your nutritional needs. But getting more vitamin D could be an easy way to improve your mental health.

For more information about vitamin D, please see "Beat disease with the sunshine vitamin" on page 82 in *Cardio health: fit for life*.

Surprising strategies sharpen your memory

Sometimes less is more. That could be the case with calories and your memory. On the other hand, sometimes more is better. Boosting your intake of water and antioxidant vitamins may give your memory a boost. Here are some surprising ways to improve your memory.

Eat less for a sharper mind. In a recent German study, overweight elderly people who cut their calories by 30 percent didn't just lose weight — they also significantly improved their memories and thinking skills. The boost was likely due to reduced insulin resistance and inflammation, which may contribute to age-related mental decline. While eating less may help you remember more, it's important to get adequate nutrition and maintain a healthy body weight as you age.

Water your brain. Like a plant, your brain needs plenty of water to flourish. If you become dehydrated, you may suffer from poor short-term memory and have difficulty learning or focusing. In fact, dehydration that results in the loss of as little as 1 percent of your body weight can have a negative impact on your mental performance. Many experts recommend drinking about eight 8-ounce glasses of water daily, but you may need more if you're exercising or dealing with high temperatures.

Vanquish fat with vitamins. A high-fat meal does more than make your pants uncomfortable. For older people with diabetes, it can also impair your memory. Luckily, high does of vitamins C and E may help, according to a recent Canadian study. Type 2 diabetes causes oxidative stress, and high-fat meals trigger even more. But antioxidant vitamins stifle memory-damaging free radicals to minimize this effect. People in the study took 1,000 milligrams (mg) of vitamin C and 800 international units (IU) of vitamin E with their meals. But you can help protect your memory by avoiding high-fat meals and eating foods rich in vitamins C and E.

Energize your brain with breakfast

Start your day the right way — with a healthy breakfast. This important meal can fight fatigue and stress, brighten your mood, and sharpen your focus and concentration. Go from exhausted to exhilarated with these tips for beating fatigue. If you always feel tired, don't miss breakfast. Just follow these six tips for morning meals that make you merry.

Wake up and smell the coffee. Caffeine can give you a jolt of energy to get you moving in the morning, but just the smell of coffee may help with stress. In a study of sleep-deprived rats, the aroma of roasted coffee beans changed the levels of some brain proteins, indicating antioxidant function and a calming effect on stress. Drink coffee and you may also reduce your risk of depression.

Get serious about cereal. In one study, people who regularly ate cereal felt less depressed, less stressed, and had lower levels of emotional distress than those who did not eat breakfast every day. Your best bet is a whole-grain, high-fiber cereal. A high fiber intake has been linked to less fatigue and emotional distress and fewer mental difficulties.

Count on carbs. Tired and sluggish? Carbohydrates will give you more energy. That's because your body breaks down carbohydrates into glucose, your body's main source of fuel. Aim for a mix of complex and simple carbohydrates. Complex carbs, including whole grains and starchy vegetables like potatoes, take longer for your body to absorb, so you get a steady stream of energy.

Simple carbs, on the other hand, give you a quick and fleeting energy boost. Fruit and honey, which contain the sugar fructose, are healthy examples of simple carbs. To get both complex and simple carbs into your breakfast, add some fruit to your whole-grain cereal. This fruity, high-fiber breakfast is a great way to keep your energy up throughout a busy morning.

Carbohydrates also affect your mood. In a Japanese study, men who ate the most carbohydrates were much less likely to show symptoms of depression than those who ate the least. A high intake of carbohydrates helps deliver the amino acid tryptophan to your brain, which stimulates the synthesis of serotonin, the brain's feel-good chemical.

Plate up some protein. For endurance, you should also include protein along with your carbohydrates. Protein helps regulate your body's release of energy. Good sources include eggs, meat, and low-fat dairy products.

Boost your B's. Low levels of B vitamins such as folate and B12 have been linked to depression. Enriched breads and cereals provide folate, while meats, dairy foods, and eggs give you vitamin B12.

Add some antioxidants. Japanese researchers found that older men who ate lots of foods rich in vitamin C and carotenoids — including beta carotene, the plant form of vitamin A — had fewer depressive symptoms than those who ate the least. These antioxidant vitamins could protect your brain from oxidative stress, which contributes to depression. Citrus fruits and other brightly colored fruits and vegetables should do the trick.

Combine some of these nutrients into a healthy breakfast. Try a whole-grain bagel with cheese, oatmeal with raisins, or whole-grain toast with peanut butter and fruit. Or enjoy scrambled eggs, toast, and fruit or hard-boiled eggs sliced in a whole-wheat pita.

Smarter ways to enjoy soy

There's good news and bad news when it comes to soy and your brain. Too much tofu may harm your memory, but other forms of soy could help save it.

Trim the tofu. A recent British study of 719 older Indonesian people found that high tofu consumption was associated with memory loss. The phytoestrogens in tofu could be the problem. Phytoestrogens, or plant estrogens, mimic the estrogen produced naturally in your body. Studies have shown that estrogen therapy doubles the risk of dementia in women over age 65.

The results echo those of a previous long-term Hawaiian study that found a higher risk of dementia, more brain shrinkage, and worse brain function in people who ate tofu more than twice a week. Researchers also pointed out that toxins could be to blame. In Indonesia, formaldehyde may be added to tofu to preserve its freshness.

Consider the alternatives. In the same study, high consumption of tempe — a fermented whole soybean product — was related to better memory. Like tofu, tempe has high phytoestrogen levels. But because it's fermented, it's also high in folate, which could help offset the negative effects.

Natto, a fermented food made from boiled soybeans and eaten for more than 1,000 years in Asia, could also provide some protection. An enzyme in natto called nattokinase does the trick. In lab tests, nattokinase dissolved blood clots and amyloid fibrils, the clumps of tangled proteins involved in Alzheimer's disease.

There are some drawbacks to natto. It may be hard to find in the United States — and it may be harder to enjoy. With its strong smell and slimy texture, it's definitely an acquired taste.

Think moderation. Besides its effect on your brain, too much soy may cause other problems, including slowed thyroid function and a higher risk of breast cancer for older women. But many health experts think eating tofu and other forms of soy in moderation should not be a problem. Just don't go overboard.

Low-carb diet starves your brain

Cutting carbohydrates to cut weight? You may also cut into your memory. A recent Tufts University study found that women in the early stages of a low-carbohydrate diet, when they eliminated all carbs, fared worse on memory tests than women sticking to a low-calorie balanced diet. That's likely because they had very low levels of glucose, your brain's main fuel. Your body breaks down carbohydrates into glucose. When the women reintroduced a small amount of carbs into their diet, their memories returned to normal.

Dietary do's and don'ts for Parkinson's

Iron man may be a popular superhero, but iron isn't so super when it comes to Parkinson's disease. Too much iron — especially from plant sources — may boost your risk. Surprisingly, foods that raise your risk for gout may lower your risk of developing Parkinson's. Remember these tips to prevent this condition.

Keep an eye on iron intake. In a recent study, Italian researchers found that people with high intakes of nonheme iron, or iron from plant sources rather than meat, had a 30 percent higher risk of Parkinson's than those who ate the least. If they also had a low intake of vitamin C, the risk jumped to 92 percent higher.

Iron could contribute to Parkinson's by increasing oxidative damage in the brain. Nonheme iron, which your body does not absorb easily, can accumulate in your brain. Previous studies have found more iron deposits in brain regions affected by Parkinson's. The main sources of nonheme iron include fortified cereals and grains.

Get wise to uric acid. A Harvard study found that foods that increase blood levels of uric acid, the compound linked to gout, reduced the risk of Parkinson's. Similarly, Canadian researchers reported that older people with gout were 30 percent less likely to develop Parkinson's. Uric acid may protect your brain's neurons from oxidative stress with its antioxidant properties. Foods that boost uric acid include anchovies, herring, mackerel, mussels, organ meats, gravy, and alcohol. Just remember that eating these foods may increase your risk of developing gout.

Brew some coffee or tea. If you really like coffee, you'll really like this news about Parkinson's disease. According to a Finnish study, drinking 10 cups a day can slash your risk by a whopping 84 percent. The caffeine in coffee may stimulate dopamine, a brain chemical lacking in people who have the disease.

Just as with coffee, more tea means more protection from Parkinson's disease. A Chinese study found that people who drank at least 23 cups of black tea a month had a 71 percent lower risk of developing Parkinson's disease than those who drank less. While caffeine was also associated with a lower risk of Parkinson's, black tea's other ingredients — including its complex antioxidants — seem to provide the protection. In animal tests, the polyphenols found in green tea also show promise for fighting Parkinson's.

Eat more vitamin E foods. A diet rich in this antioxidant vitamin could protect you from Parkinson's, according to a Canadian study. Opt for vitamin E from food sources, such as green leafy vegetables, seeds, nuts, and olive oil, rather than supplements.

Beware of protein. Dietary protein can interfere with levodopa, a common drug for Parkinson's. You can improve the medication's effectiveness by taking it 45 minutes before meals with a cracker. You may also want to limit your protein intake during the day.

Other natural remedies

Rethink ginkgo as memory aid

There are two sides to every story, and ginkgo is no exception.
While ginkgo has long been considered a valuable memory-boosting
supplement, recent studies have cast doubt on its effectiveness.
Find out more about this ancient herb and how it may — or may
not — give your brain a boost.

Gloomy outlook. One recent study of people age 85 or older in
Oregon found that taking the supplement had no clear-cut benefit
on the risk of developing memory problems. Even worse, there was
an increased risk for stroke and transient ischemic attack (TIA), or
mini-stroke, among those who took ginkgo.

A bigger study called Ginkgo Evaluation of Memory (GEM),
which followed more than 3,000 people age 75 or older for an
average of six years, showed ginkgo was no help in preventing
dementia, including Alzheimer's. This study also came with more
bad news — those with heart disease when the study started actually increased their risk for dementia by 56 percent.

Ginkgo comes with some other concerns. It may interact danger-
ously with blood-thinning drugs, such as aspirin or warfarin. Avoid
ginkgo if you have bleeding disorders or if you've had a stroke.
Stop taking ginkgo two weeks before planned surgery to avoid an
increased risk of bleeding. A few people may experience side
effects like nervousness, headache, and stomachache if they take
high doses of ginkgo.

Glimmer of hope. But not all the news about ginkgo is bad. Even
in the recent less-than-positive studies, poor adherence may have
played a role. In the Oregon study, those who followed directions

and reliably took the supplement had a 68 percent lower risk of developing mild dementia. By the end of the GEM study, only 60 percent of the participants were taking their assigned medications, which may have skewed the outcome.

Several earlier studies yielded positive results, especially for people in the early stages of dementia. One study even found ginkgo to be as effective as the drug Aricept — with fewer side effects. Even in people without memory problems, ginkgo improved short-term memory and concentration in several studies.

Ginkgo may work by increasing blood flow to the brain. Restricted blood and oxygen flow could be a factor in the development of Alzheimer's. The herb may also help by increasing the activity of acetylcholine, a neurotransmitter essential for short-term memory.

Weigh the pros and cons of ginkgo, taking into account your current health, and talk to your doctor before taking any supplements. If you decide to try ginkgo, look for products containing ginkgo biloba leaf extract (GBE) with 24 percent flavonol glycosides. Standard dosage varies from 120 milligrams (mg) to 240 mg daily.

Little-known brain boosters worth remembering

Some supplements fly under the radar — but that doesn't make them any less powerful. Keep these little-known supplements in mind to give your memory a lift.

Bacopa monnieri. This creeping herb that grows in marshy areas of India, Australia, and the tropics has potent antioxidant properties and helps reduce oxidative stress. Lab tests in Thailand showed it protected brain cells from cell death caused by beta-amyloids, proteins that form plaques in the brain, which are thought to contribute to Alzheimer's. This makes it a promising alternative treatment for Alzheimer's disease and other brain disorders.

A 12-week study in Oregon found that 300 milligrams (mg) of *bacopa monnieri* a day helped older people improve on memory and learning tests. It also lowered depression and anxiety. *Bacopa monnieri* may work by improving nerve function in the brain's hippocampus, an important site for memory.

Huperzine A. This chemical purified from leaves of the Chinese toothed club moss can also be synthetically manufactured. Three Chinese studies including more than 450 people found that huperzine A improved symptoms of Alzheimer's disease and other forms of dementia. Its positive effects on memory, thinking, and behavior in people with dementia make this supplement worthy of the "A" in its name.

Like some prescription drugs used to treat Alzheimer's, huperzine A works by blocking the breakdown of the neurotransmitter acetylcholine, which is essential for short-term memory.

For Alzheimer's, doses range from 50 to 200 micrograms (mcg) twice daily. As a bonus, huperzine A may enhance the effects of prescription drugs, like Aricept or Cognex, so you can lower your dosage and experience fewer side effects. Use with caution if you have heart problems, because it can decrease your heart rate.

Gotu kola. Like *bacopa monnieri*, this ancient herb has long been used as an alternative medicine for memory enhancement in Ayurvedic medicine. Studies suggest it may also help with anxiety. In several studies, gotu kola lessened mental impairment in rats with Alzheimer's. Researchers working with rats recently pinpointed a possible molecular mechanism for its memory-boosting properties. While it's not clear if gotu kola works for people, it certainly shows promise.

Rejuvenate your brain with Juvenon

Boxers who throw combinations generally have more success than those who throw only one punch at a time. Take the same approach with supplements. Give your brain a one-two jolt with the powerful combination of acetyl-L-carnitine and alpha lipoic acid. Available together in the supplement Juvenon, these compounds boost your energy and your brain.

Acetyl-L-carnitine is an amino acid believed to play a role in the production of acetylcholine, an important neurotransmitter. Lipoic acid acts as an antioxidant. While your body naturally synthesizes both substances, you can also get them through food.

Together, they have a positive effect on your mitochondria, the tiny powerhouses in your cells that burn food for fuel. Changes in mito-chondria that occur over a lifetime may play a key role in aging, and weakened mitochondria may leave people more susceptible to Parkinson's disease or speed up the progression of Alzheimer's. Acetyl-L-carnitine delivers fat to your mitochondria to be burned as fuel, while lipoic acid protects your mitochondria from free radical damage.

Although human studies of Juvenon are still in the works, results of animal studies have been promising. In one study, old, sedentary rats spontaneously doubled their physical activity. In another, old rats had less mitochondrial damage in their brains and performed better on memory tasks than rats given a placebo. The supplement also improved short-term memory and learning in beagles.

Each Juvenon tablet includes 500 milligrams (mg) of carnitine and 200 mg of lipoic acid, but animal studies used very high doses. You can order Juvenon online at *www.juvenon.com* or by calling 800-567-2502.

Dodge dangerous drug interactions

St. John's wort may work as well as some prescription drugs — but it doesn't always work well with them. Beware of interactions. This herb can weaken the power of many medications, including cholesterol-lowering drugs, blood pressure drugs, and blood thinners.

If you take St. John's wort along with selective serotonin reuptake inhibitors (SSRIs), such as Prozac or Zoloft, it may trigger a dangerous condition called serotonin syndrome. You might become confused, hot, sweaty, and restless and experience headaches, stomachaches, muscle spasms, or seizures.

Natural way to defeat depression

Looking for a safe, natural alternative to prescription antidepressants? Look no further than St. John's wort. This herbal remedy can lift your mood without unpleasant side effects.

Several clinical trials and reviews of studies have determined that St. John's wort works better than a placebo, or dummy pill, and just as well as prescription antidepressants — including Prozac and Zoloft — for mild to moderate depression.

But the news may be even better. In a recent review of 29 studies, German researchers concluded that St. John's wort may work as well as prescription antidepressants for major depression, too. In one six-week study comparing St. John's wort to paroxetine (Paxil), those taking St. John's wort improved their depression scores by 57 percent, while those taking paroxetine improved by only 45 percent — and were more likely to experience side effects, like dry mouth, dizziness, nausea, and diarrhea.

St. John's wort likely gets its powers from the active ingredients hypericin and hyperforin. It may work by inhibiting the reuptake of the neurotransmitters serotonin, dopamine, and noradrenaline. This means that, rather than being reabsorbed and recycled by the cells that originally produced them, these chemicals remain in the brain to boost your mood.

Standard dosage is 900 milligrams (mg) daily, divided into two or three doses. It may take two to four weeks to notice any improvement.

Smile more with SAM-e

A popular supplement for osteoarthritis does more than soothe your joints. It also helps brighten your mood. S-adenosyl-methionine, better known as SAM-e, can be a safe way to combat depression.

SAM-e, a natural compound found in every cell of your body, has antioxidant and anti-inflammatory powers. It even helps in the production of brain chemicals called neurotransmitters, such as serotonin and dopamine. Its influence on neurotransmitter metabolism, membrane fluidity, and receptor activity could explain its antidepressant effect.

In a recent 30-person study, Harvard researchers found that SAM-e helped some severely depressed people who did not respond to traditional medications. When they added SAM-e to standard antidepressants such as Zoloft or Effexor, they got response rates of 40 to 50 percent. Unlike some standard antidepressants, SAM-e does not cause weight gain or sexual dysfunction.

Earlier short-term studies showed that SAM-e works better than a placebo and just as well as tricyclics, a class of older antidepressants, in treating depression. Studies are underway to test SAM-e against newer drugs, such as selective serotonin reuptake inhibitors (SSRIs).

Doses range from 400 milligrams (mg) to 1,600 mg a day. Cost can range from $18 to $50 or more a month. To avoid possible nausea or upset stomach, look for SAM-e supplements with enteric coating. Unless you're following your doctor's advice, do not take SAM-e with other antidepressants. If you have bipolar disorder, SAM-e may trigger a manic phase.

2 ways to ease anxiety and depression

Whether you need to fall asleep or stay awake, you can find an herbal remedy. Valerian fights insomnia, while goldenroot battles fatigue. Both herbs may also help combat anxiety and depression.

Valerian. Known as a sleep aid, valerian may also come in handy for relief of anxiety. Although there have been few studies, they have been encouraging. Valerian helped people with generalized anxiety disorder in one study, and improved measures of stress — like systolic blood pressure, heart rate, and self-reported stress — in another. In one study of people with depression and anxiety, those who took valerian along with St. John's wort fared better than those who took St. John's wort alone.

Valerian may work by affecting the activity of the neurotransmitter GABA in the central nervous system, the target of most prescription tranquilizers and sleep aids. The usual dose is 400 to 600 milligrams (mg) a day. Keep in mind that it may take several weeks to work.

Goldenroot. Often used to treat chronic fatigue, goldenroot may also help lift your mood. A Swedish study found that it reduced symptoms of depression in people with mild to moderate depression. It also improved their mental function. An Armenian study of people with mild to moderate depression showed that goldenroot improved overall depression, as well as insomnia and emotional instability, with no serious side effects. Dosage was either 340 or 680 mg a day over six weeks.

Also known as *Rhodiola rosea*, goldenroot boasts anti-stress powers, too. It has helped fatigued doctors perform under stressful conditions and countered the effects of stress-induced anorexia in rats. It works by normalizing levels of brain chemicals that affect mood to help counter the effects of stress.

Healthful living

Escape depression and dementia with a little help from your friends

You could live up to 22 percent longer just by having more friends. Socializing helps extend your life, fight depression, and ward off dementia. In an Australian study, older people with the largest network of good friends were more likely to survive during the 10-year follow-up period. In fact, those with the most friends were 22 percent less likely to die than those with the least. Researchers suspect friends may encourage older people to take better care of themselves. They may also help you get through tough times, boosting your mood and self-esteem. So make more friends, and make the most of your life.

Just be sure they're happy friends. A University of California San Diego study found that happiness is contagious. People surrounded by many happy people are more likely to become happy. If a friend who lives within a mile of you becomes happy, your odds of becoming happy increase by 25 percent. Researchers found similar effects for spouses, siblings who lived within a mile, and next-door neighbors.

Friends not only spread happiness, they can also sharpen your mind. In a recent study of 2,249 women age 78 or older, those with larger social networks had a 26 percent lower risk of dementia compared to those with smaller networks of friends and family members.

You may not need a large circle of friends. Maintaining relationships with small groups of close friends or family members can also keep your mind sharp. Remember, social interactions don't always have to be face to face. You can keep in touch by phone, e-mail, or letters.

Even talking helps. A University of Michigan study found that having a 10-minute conversation was just as effective as doing an intellectual activity in terms of boosting memory and mental performance. That means just visiting a neighbor or friend can be just as helpful in keeping your brain sharp as doing a daily crossword puzzle. So can playing bridge, which combines mental activity with social interaction.

Romantic relationships also matter. An interesting recent study suggests that people who are unmarried or living alone during midlife may have an increased risk of developing Alzheimer's disease. Those who were married or lived with a significant other during midlfe had a 50 percent lower risk of developing dementia later in life.

Unexpected benefit for caregivers

Taking care of your husband or wife not only helps your spouse — it may also help you live longer. A recent University of Michigan study found that older people who spent at least 14 hours a week caring for a disabled spouse lived longer than those who provided no spousal care.

Prayer keeps you out of a nursing home

Practice that old-time religion, and you may spend less time in a long-term care facility. A Duke University study showed that religious beliefs and spirituality make a difference in how many days of long-term care you need.

Specifically, the study focused on praying and reading the Bible, tuning into religious radio or television programs, and daily spiritual experiences. Seniors who do these kind of activities are the least likely to need care in nursing homes or rehab centers. During the study, those who participated in these activities the most had significantly shorter stays than those who did them the least. The effect was strongest among blacks and women.

All of these activities were also associated with greater social support, which could be a key factor. Another explanation is that religious people come from religious families, who may be more likely to take care of loved ones rather than rely on a nursing home. Religion may also provide hope and motivate you to do more things for yourself, delaying the need for long-term care.

Religious or spiritual activities have been linked to better physical and mental health and a longer life. Praying may be good for your mind and body as well as your soul. Amen.

Better to give than to receive

Being generous with your money can make you happier. A recent study found that people who spent money on gifts and charity were happier than those who spent it on themselves. Just spending $5 on others can improve your mood.

Watch the scale to preserve your mind

Maintaining a healthy weight may help you maintain a healthy mind. Studies show that paying attention to the scale may pay off later in life. Dutch researchers reviewed seven previous studies and found that being overweight significantly increases your risk of dementia. People age 65 and older who were obese at the start of the studies were 80 percent more likely to develop dementia.

A Johns Hopkins review of 10 international studies from the United States, Finland, Sweden, France, and Japan reached a similar conclusion. Obese people have an 80 percent greater risk of Alzheimer's disease compared to those with normal weight. Ages ranged from 40 to 80 when the studies started, and follow-up lasted from three to 36 years. Just don't go overboard with dieting. Being underweight also poses a risk, making you 36 percent more likely to develop dementia. The key is to maintain a healthy weight.

Where your fat is located also makes a difference. One recent study found that having a big belly during middle age gives you a bigger risk of dementia later in life. Those with the most abdominal fat were nearly three times more likely to develop dementia than those with the least. Even those with a normal weight, but a big belly, were at added risk.

Read on to discover fun and easy ways to shed pounds and keep your body — and mind — in shape.

Simply amazing way to keep your brain in shape

You can really help your brain think better, remember more, and stay young longer. It doesn't cost anything, and you can start today. What's more, you'll see the benefits right away. Just start moving. Exercise has a tremendous effect on your brain. This 100 percent natural solution does it all. Grow new brain cells, stop high blood pressure, and keep your brain from shrinking.

Reverse your brain's age. A recent University of Illinois study found that aerobic exercise helps halt — and even reverse — brain shrinkage in healthy older people. People in the six-month study increased their brains' volume of both gray matter, or neurons, and white matter, the connections between the neurons, in areas of the brain that often show age-related deterioration.

It took just three months for these people to boost their brain volume to what it was three years earlier, according to lead researcher Arthur Kramer. And they did it with one easy exercise — three hours a week of brisk walking.

Exercise may help by improving blood flow to the brain, leading to an increase in neurotransmitters and the birth of new brain cells. Regular exercise also helps keep arteries elastic to ensure normal blood flow, protecting you against high blood pressure and stroke.

Cut your risk of dementia. A daily 30-minute walk could be all it takes to boost your brain. In a study of older Italian men and women, those who took a brisk walk more often saw their risk of dementia drop 27 percent, compared to the people who walked the least. An Australian study of people with memory problems found that physical activity, including walking, led to a modest improvement.

It's not just aerobic exercises that help. There's also evidence that resistance training, such as weight lifting, provides benefits for your brain.

Another study suggests that regular exercise can delay the onset of Alzheimer's and other forms of dementia. Compared to those who exercised fewer than three times a week, older people who exercised three or more times a week cut their risk of dementia, including Alzheimer's disease, by 30 to 40 percent. All because of what they did three times a week.

A Mayo Clinic study found that moderate exercise that took place between ages 50 and 65 may reduce the risk of mild impairment in your thinking processes, which often progresses to Alzheimer's, later in life.

Even if you already have Alzheimer's, exercise may help. One study found that less physically fit people with Alzheimer's had four times the brain shrinkage of those in better shape. People in the early stages of Alzheimer's may be able to preserve brain function longer by exercising regularly.

Stay active. Not only will it help you live a longer, healthier life, it could even determine where you spend your golden years. Regular exercise could help you stay sharp, sidestep Alzheimer's disease, and avoid life in a nursing home.

Wii works wonders for seniors

You don't have to be a couch potato to play video games. Have fun — and get some exercise — with Nintendo Wii. This easy-to-use gaming system is becoming a hit with seniors. And it's easy to see why.

Unlike most video games, which have complicated controls, Wii uses a handheld motion-sensitive controller. You just mimic familiar actions to play virtual sports, such as tennis, bowling, baseball, and golf. It's a great way to boost hand-eye coordination, improve your balance, and make exercise more fun. It also encourages socialization, another big benefit for your brain. Just don't get carried away and forget your physical limitations. The Wii system costs about $250 — but its effect on your brain could be priceless.

Powerful way to fight depression

Exercise doesn't just improve your memory — it can also improve your mood. Physical activity is a natural and powerful way to fight depression. You don't need to join a gym, run, or lift weights. Simply walking can do the trick. A study of 380 menopausal women in Philadelphia found that brisk walking can help lower stress, anxiety, and depression. People in the study walked at a moderate pace for an hour and a half five days a week.

Even 20 minutes of housework can help — as long as you work up a sweat. A British study determined that both housecleaning and walking lowered the risk of depression by 20 percent. Gardening slashed the risk of depression by 24 percent. The key to any activity is that it must be for 20 minutes at a time and make you feel breathless.

Exercise may help by curbing biological risk factors for depression, such as glucose intolerance, inflammation, and cardiovascular problems. On the other hand, those who suffer from stress and anxiety may be less likely to exercise in the first place. Depression often leads to a decrease in energy and motivation. It may be tough to motivate yourself to start moving — but you'll be amazed by how well you feel after exercising.

Even if you don't lose weight, exercise can help improve your mood and emotional health, according to a Louisiana State University study. Regular exercise can also improve the quality of life for inactive, overweight older women.

Fresh air might help, too. British researchers found that people were happier, less tense, and had more energy after taking a walk outside compared to walking inside.

Surprising strategy to keep your mind sharp

Keeping your blood pressure and blood sugar under control helps you avoid health problems like stroke and diabetes. But it may also help keep your mind sharp as you age.

Ease the pressure. High blood pressure isn't just a key risk factor for stroke. When you have high blood pressure, you're 600 times more likely to develop vascular dementia. High blood pressure restricts oxygen to the brain, but symptoms often go unnoticed. A Howard University study found a similar link. In people age 70 or older, high blood pressure was associated with worse mental function than normal blood pressure. According to the Alzheimer's Society, high blood pressure also doubles your risk of another type of dementia — Alzheimer's disease.

If you want to keep your wits about you as you age, take steps to lower your blood pressure — and your risk of dementia. Make sure to get your blood pressure checked regularly. You can also help yourself by sticking to a healthy diet low in sodium and high in potassium, exercising regularly, maintaining a healthy weight, limiting your alcohol intake, quitting smoking, and managing stress.

Get smart about sugar. High blood sugar puts you at high risk for diabetes. It's not so sweet for your memory, either. A new Columbia University study found that rising blood sugar levels may be partly responsible for lapses in memory. Researchers found a link between rising blood sugar levels and decreasing activity in the dentate gyrus, a part of the brain's hippocampus critical for memory. Lowering blood sugar should boost dentate gyrus function and help your brain.

A long-term study of men in Sweden found that those who develop diabetes in midlife are more likely to develop Alzheimer's in old age. Diabetes was also linked to impairment in thought processes, which often precedes Alzheimer's. As with diabetes, insulin resistance may play a role in the development of Alzheimer's. Exercise may be a good way to keep your blood sugar under control.

Action plan for people with memory problems

Early diagnosis is key when it comes to Alzheimer's disease. But too often, people deny or cover up symptoms. This only delays treatment — perhaps until it's too late. Current drugs only slow the progression of Alzheimer's, so you need to catch it before it becomes more severe.

An early diagnosis also lets you participate in making treatment decisions while you still can. It's also important to rule out memory problems from other causes, such as depression, thyroid problems, vitamin deficiencies, and side effects from certain medications. Diagnosis should include a complete physical with lab tests and MRI, as well as mental tests. You'll get the most accurate diagnosis at centers that specialize in Alzheimer's disease or geriatrics.

Memory-boosting tricks you'll never forget

Ever forget someone's name right after you met them? How embarrassing! Make sure that doesn't happen again with these sure-fire tips for perfect name recall.

- Focus on the name. Paying attention is important. Listen closely when someone introduces himself. Look directly at the person to eliminate distractions.

- Repeat it. After someone tells you his name, repeat it. "Nice to meet you, Carl." Saying the name impresses it into your memory more than just hearing it. You can also make a comment about the name. "My best friend growing up was named Carl."

- Spell it. If you need reinforcement, ask how to spell it. "Is that Carl with a C or a K?"

- Visualize it. Create a visual image to make a person's name more vivid and easier to remember. For instance, if you meet a Mr. Waters, picture him swimming.

- Associate it. Some names can be associated with something about the person. Maybe you think Lilah smells like lilacs, or Julie is wearing an interesting jewel on a necklace.

- Use it. Once you know someone's name, use it frequently in your conversation to keep it fixed in your mind.

Of course, you may have problems remembering things other than names. If you often misplace items, like your car keys, make a habit of always putting them in the same spot. Or act like a sports announcer and give a play-by-play of your actions. "I'm putting the keys on the table."

Maybe you need to remember a short list of things to do. Try singing your list to the tune of a familiar song or making an acronym out of your list. You can also use an odd reminder — like placing a shoe on that stack of unpaid bills on your desk. You'll notice something out of place, then realize what you're supposed to do.

Ever have a word on the tip of your tongue? Go through the alphabet. When you get to the letter it starts with, it should trigger your memory.

If all else fails, the best thing to do may be to forget about it. Instead of wracking your brain to remember a word or name, just relax. Concentrating too hard could make it worse. Take a break, do something else, and let the unconscious side of your brain work on it. The answer may come to you out of the blue.

7 super strategies to save your brain

Use it or lose it. That's the key to keeping your brain in tiptop shape. Try these tactics to improve your memory and ward off dementia.

Change things up. Use different parts of your brain to do familiar tasks. For example, brush your teeth with your nondominant hand or shower with your eyes closed. Take a different route to work or switch the usual seating arrangements at the dinner table. Novelty helps spark new brain cells and connections between them.

Choose stimulating hobbies. A recent study found that certain activities may delay or prevent memory loss. Reading books, playing games, engaging in computer activities, and doing crafts like pottery and quilting led to a 30 to 50 percent decrease in the risk of developing memory loss compared to people who did not do these things.

Turn off the TV. The same study found that older people who watch television for less than seven hours a day are half as likely to develop memory loss as those who watch it for more than seven hours a day.

Learn more languages. A Tel Aviv University study found that knowing and speaking many languages may protect your brain from the effects of aging. Speaking more languages means you're likely to be clear-minded at an older age. Languages may create new links in the brain.

Work less. All work and no play could lead to decreased mental function. In a Finnish study of British civil servants, those who worked more than 55 hours a week had poorer mental skills, including short-term memory and recall, compared to those who worked no more than 40 hours a week.

Sidestep secondhand smoke. University of Cambridge researchers found that secondhand smoke increases your odds of mental impairment. They measured salivary cotinine concentration, a bio-marker of exposure to secondhand smoke. Those with the highest concentration were at 44 percent greater risk.

Take on challenges. The important thing is to give your brain a workout. Solve crossword or Sudoku puzzles, play board or card games, test new recipes, take a class, travel to unfamiliar places, or try hobbies that force you to learn new skills.

High-tech ways to spark your brain power

You may think surfing the Internet and playing video games are activities reserved for your teenage grandchildren. But these high-tech pastimes may improve your brain function as you get older.

A recent UCLA study found that performing Web searches stimulates and possibly improves brain function in middle-age and older adults. Surprisingly, searching the Web may be even more helpful than reading because it triggers more activity in the areas of the brain that control decision making and complex reasoning.

When searching the Web, you need to make decisions on what to click to find more information. Both reading and Web searching boosted activity in regions of the brain controlling language, reading, memory, and visual abilities.

Just as with any new activity, practice makes perfect. Those with Internet experience showed much more brain activity than those with limited experience. So you may want to bone up on your Web surfing skills.

You may also want to start playing video games. A recent University of Illinois study found that older people who played a complex video game after receiving training improved on tests of memory and reasoning. They also were better able to juggle multiple tasks, which could come in handy in day-to-day life. Researchers note that you might want to play with other people, so you don't miss out on the benefits of social interaction.

You can even go to a "brain gym" to work out. Instead of lifting weights or running on a treadmill, you sit at a computer station with "mental fitness" software. Like other gyms, these facilities charge a fee. You may also be able to find a similar setup in community centers and retirement communities. Of course, you can also play games and do brain-teasing puzzles for free online.

Snooze your way to a sharper mind

You would get fired for sleeping on the job — but that's when your brain does some of its best work. Your body has hormones that repair it and slow down the aging process — it's their job. But our modern lifestyle can interfere. Discover how to naturally stimulate your body to release more of these tireless workers, for a sharper mind and more youthful feeling and appearance.

Recharge with super sleep benefits. Several studies have shown the powerful effect sleep has on your brain. Sleep boosts procedural memory, which helps you remember how to perform certain actions,

and declarative memory, or the ability to recall facts and events —
as well as short-term memory.

As you sleep, your brain replays information over and over to consolidate the memory over time. Sleep may even help produce new brain cells. Rats deprived of sleep produce fewer new brain cells in the hippocampus, an area of the brain important for long-term memory.

Even naps can help. A few studies found that people remembered things they'd just learned better if they napped afterward. Naps as short as six minutes can help your memory. As soon as you doze off, your brain goes to work, sorting memories into those you need for long-term and short-term recall and discarding the rest.

That's why your long-term memory can actually get better as you age. Just make sure to get enough quality sleep.

Sleeping also helps your skin cells regenerate more quickly. Lose just a few hours of sleep, and you may end up with dark circles under your eyes. Frequent sleep deprivation can lead to dry, dull skin all over your body.

Take steps for better sleep. If you want to improve your memory and your skin, try improving your sleep. Here are some simple tips to help you sleep soundly.

- Stick to a regular sleep schedule.

- Exercise regularly, but do vigorous exercise early in the day.

- Avoid coffee and other sources of caffeine after midmorning.

- Pass on heavy meals too close to bedtime.

- Cut down or eliminate alcohol.

- Use your bed only for sleep or sex. Watch TV or read elsewhere.

- Do not try to sleep when you're not tired.

- Get treatment for conditions that can lead to sleep problems, such as depression, anxiety, sleep apnea, and restless legs syndrome.

- Use sleeping pills only as a last resort.

- Ask your doctor if side effects from your medications may interfere with your sleep.

You may also want to limit watching TV or using a computer in the evening. A Japanese study found that people who did those things for more than three hours a night were more likely to report insufficient sleep. Using a cell phone before bed may also disrupt your natural sleep rhythms.

Discover how light can help your brain

Shine a bright light in your living room, and you may slow dementia and fight depression. In a Dutch study, installing bright lights in the common living areas of nursing homes lessened mental decline by 5 percent, reduced depression symptoms by 19 percent, and slowed the gradual increase in daily living limitations by 53 percent.

Researchers note that your body's circadian timing system plays a role in optimal brain health, and disturbances in this rhythm often occur in older people and those with dementia. Exposure to light can gradually help get your body's daily clock back on track.

Bright light also helps combat seasonal affective disorder, or SAD, a form of depression that occurs during the diminished daylight hours of late fall and winter. A recent Austrian study determined a link between SAD and low levels of serotonin, a mood-regulating brain chemical. In people with SAD, a protein that helps transport serotonin does its job too well, snatching serotonin from the bloodstream — where it's available — and moving it to the platelets, where it's not. After beneficial light therapy, the protein slows down, allowing more serotonin to remain in the bloodstream. It may work the same way in the brain.

To make the most of light, go outside at the same time each day. You should also avoid bright light within three hours of bedtime. If you think you have SAD, ask your doctor about light therapy, which involves sitting for about 30 minutes in front of a lamp that uses multiple fluorescent lights.

Name that tune for a brain tune-up

You can never get some songs out of your head — and that's a good thing. Listening to music, especially familiar songs, can help slow the progression of Alzheimer's. Music also helps fight anxiety and depression.

Listen up. Listening to music can help people with Alzheimer's reconnect with their memories and rediscover their personality. It can even help you recall names, faces, and words, according to a study by the Institute for Music and Neurologic Function in New York. If you have dementia, familiar tunes can help you relate to others and experience joy.

That's because music is powerful. Unlike verbal memory, music memory does not rest in one specific part of your brain. Since it's processed across many parts, it's harder to erase music from your mind. Not just any music will do. Songs that were popular when you were a teen or young adult have the most impact.

Sing along. Actually making music also helps. According to the British Alzheimer's Society, singing familiar songs and learning new ones can help build self-esteem and ease loneliness for people with dementia. It may even delay the onset of memory problems. One study found that moving to music, playing rhythm instruments, and singing led to more group involvement and less disruptive behavior among people with dementia in nursing facilities.

Singing in a group, such as a church choir or community chorale, also provides beneficial social ties. People with more social ties are less likely to develop mental decline.

Cheer up. According to a Cleveland Clinic study, listening to music can ease depression symptoms by 25 percent. Other studies have shown different types of music reduce levels of the stress hormone cortisol and lower blood pressure. Music can even ward off fatigue during exercise. A South Korean study found that music can improve depression, anxiety, and relationships in people with mental illness.

Medical alternatives

Quick new tests detect early Alzheimer's

The number of people with Alzheimer's is growing rapidly — and rapid detection is key to treating this disease. Researchers on both sides of the Atlantic have recently designed speedy and accurate tests to detect early signs of dementia.

Emory University researchers developed a two-part screening test called MC-FAQ to flag mild cognitive impairment, often the first stage of Alzheimer's. It takes about three minutes, as opposed to 40 or 60 minutes for standard tests — and it's nearly as accurate. Mini-Cog consists of a simple clock drawing task and three-item recall. Meanwhile, a spouse or other family member completes a Functional Activities Questionnaire.

Researchers at Addenbrooke's Hospital in Cambridge, England, designed a test called TYM, or "Test Your Memory." It consists of a series of 10 tasks, including the ability to copy a sentence, knowledge of words and phrases, calculation, verbal fluency, and recall ability. Not only is TYM faster than standard tests, it's also more accurate, detecting 93 percent of people with Alzheimer's compared to 52 percent for the Mini Mental State Exam, the most commonly used test to determine mental status. This could make TYM a better tool for catching early Alzheimer's disease.

Neither test requires special training to administer. With the number of new cases of Alzheimer's expected to increase by half a million a year, these new tests could come in handy by making it quicker and easier to detect this disease.

Injection of hope for people with essential tremor

As many as one in five people over age 65 may have essential tremor (ET), a neurological condition that involves involuntary muscle contractions, usually in your hands. You may experience tremor either when your body is held in certain positions (postural tremor) or while performing an action, like writing or eating (kinetic tremor). Older people with ET often have dementia, too.

One study found that Botox injections in the wrist helped reduce postural tremor — but the injections could lead to weakness in your hands. Botox, or botulinum toxin type A, helps control muscle hyperactivity. Ask your doctor about this potential treatment.

New role for cold sore treatment

Anti-viral drugs used to treat cold sores may also help prevent Alzheimer's disease. That's because the herpes virus that causes cold sores can also trigger the protein plaques that accumulate in the brains of people with Alzheimer's.

University of Manchester researchers found DNA evidence of herpes simplex virus type 1 in 90 percent of plaques in the brains of people with Alzheimer's. They suspect the virus enters the brains of older people as their immune system declines, then remains dormant until it's activated by stress or other infections. It damages brain cells, which die and disintegrate, releasing the proteins that develop into amyloid plaques. This promising research suggests anti-viral drugs may treat Alzheimer's and raises the possibility of vaccination to prevent it.

Promising new way to fight dementia

Statins can do wonders for your heart. But these cholesterol-lowering drugs might also help protect your brain. Evidence suggests statins may help prevent Alzheimer's disease and other forms of dementia.

A University of Michigan study found that older people who took statins were about half as likely to develop dementia or mental impairment as those who didn't take them. The study, part of the Sacramento Area Latino Study on Aging, followed 1,674 Mexican Americans age 60 and older for five years.

Boston University researchers discovered that the type of statin may make a difference. In their study, which used data from the decision support system of the U.S. Veterans Affairs database, simvastatin reduced the incidence of Alzheimer's and Parkinson's disease by about 50 percent. The combination of the drug's high potency and its ability to penetrate the blood-brain barrier could be the key to its success. Statins' ability to reduce inflammation, which contributes to Alzheimer's and Parkinson's, could also play a role.

Not every study has been positive. One recent study found no relation between statin use and the risk of Alzheimer's or decline in thinking ability. A review of two major studies determined that statins worked no better than placebo. Everyone agrees more research is needed, but statins could be a very effective way to fight dementia.

Beware of memory-sapping drugs

Sometimes a solution can lead to more problems. The medications you're taking for urinary incontinence or Parkinson's disease may be harming your memory. A class of drugs called anticholinergics, also used to treat ulcers, stomach cramps, respiratory problems, and motion sickness, may cause older people to lose their thinking skills more quickly. Long known to worsen the memories of people with Alzheimer's, these drugs may also impair the memory of healthy older people, according to recent studies.

Anticholinergic drugs work by blocking the binding of the brain chemical acetylcholine to its receptor in nerve cells. But you need acetylcholine for a good memory. In fact, drugs used to treat Alzheimer's block the enzyme that breaks down acetylcholine, allowing more of it to be used by the brain.

Regular use of anticholinergics may hamper your ability to perform daily tasks, such as shopping and managing your money. The more of these drugs you take, the more your memory and ability to function declines. Older people may be more vulnerable to these drugs because of changes in the brain related to aging.

Of course, other drugs can also harm your brain. According to WorstPills.org, a consumer resource for prescription drug information, drug-induced mental impairment is most commonly linked to benzodiazepines, opiates, tricyclic antidepressants, and anticonvulsants, or anti-seizure drugs.

If you are taking one of these drugs, ask your doctor if you need to continue taking the medication. Follow his advice and never stop taking any medication without his approval.

High-tech way to fight depression

You're not alone if you're taking antidepressants — but not getting any better. Studies show 40 percent of depressed people fail to respond to antidepressants, and 70 percent do not experience a full remission. Fortunately, a new treatment may help.

A device called NeuroStar provides transcranial magnetic stimulation by delivering magnetic pulses into your skull, targeting regions of your brain involved with mood regulation. Approved by the FDA for people with major depression who have not experienced relief from antidepressant medications, NeuroStar is a noninvasive, safe, and effective prescription treatment performed in a doctor's office. Each treatment lasts about 40 minutes a day for four to six weeks. You remain awake and alert during the procedure.

For more information about NeuroStar and to locate a provider near you, go to *www.neuronetics.com* or call the Neuronetics customer service center at 877-600-7555.

Cardio health: fit for life

Super foods slash your heart disease risk

If there were a diet that could help you live five years longer and included a variety of delicious foods, wouldn't you try it? Now you can — and it's the way people in Italy and Greece have been eating for centuries.

Experts say if you build most of your meals around these fabulous foods — and avoid items not on the list, like refined sugar, white flour, and saturated fat, you'll live longer and keep your body healthy. Some of these super foods are part of the much-studied Mediterranean diet. Others are included in an eating plan called the Polymeal. The bottom line is they're all delicious and wonderfully good for you.

- fatty fish, like salmon

- fruits and vegetables

- beans

- whole-grain breads and cereals

- olive oil

- nuts, like almonds and walnuts

- dark chocolate

- grapes or red wine

- garlic and other powerful spices

You'll read more about how these foods help your heart in the stories that follow, but keep in mind how important a smart combination of foods is to your overall health. Here's what they can do for you.

Help you live five years longer. More than 300,000 AARP members took part in a study, answering questions about what they eat, how they live, and how good their health is. After five years they filled out another questionnaire. At the end of the study, people who closely followed a Mediterranean eating plan were more likely to be alive and kicking than those who didn't. This eating pattern is based on the traditional foods of Greece and southern Italy, where rates of chronic disease were low and life spans were long.

The Mediterranean diet works in the modern world, too, slashing heart attack risk by 50 percent. Among people who had already had one heart attack, those who tried to follow the plan had a 50 to 70 percent lower risk of a second heart attack or other heart event than those who ate a more traditional Western diet.

Cut heart disease risk by 76 percent. Researchers picked the top six foods in this list — fish, wine, dark chocolate, fruits and vegetables, almonds, and garlic — and called them the Polymeal. Eating these foods in abundance helps cut your heart disease risk by lowering your blood pressure and cholesterol levels, which reduces your chances of heart attack and stroke and extends your life span. That means these tasty foods help you live longer and enjoy those added years in better health.

Reduce your risk of high blood pressure. Men and women in Spain who followed a Mediterranean diet lowered their risk of age-related high blood pressure. Experts say the benefits are from polyphenols — certain natural plant compounds — in olive oil, a major ingredient in the diet. Polyphenols regulate blood pressure by keeping your arteries elastic and preventing plaques from building up on artery walls.

Help prevent Alzheimer's disease. The same anti-inflammatory and antioxidant benefits that protect your heart and blood vessels may also keep your brain young. Get lots of antioxidants by eating your share of fruits, vegetables, legumes, and nuts.

Tips on eating the Mediterranean way

You've never been to Greece or Italy, but you want to try eating like the people who live there. Here's a dinner menu based on the Mediterranean diet.

- Start with an appetizer of hummus dip, made from garbanzo beans, with whole-wheat pita bread for dipping.

- Toss up a green salad dressed with olive oil and vinegar.

- Serve broiled salmon drizzled with olive oil and sprinkled with crushed garlic.

- Steam green beans with almond slivers.

- Add a glass of purple grape juice or a single glass of red wine if you drink wine.

- Enjoy a bowl of mixed fruit topped with yogurt dressing for dessert.

Cut your chances of breast cancer. One study of various patterns of eating found that women who followed the Mediterranean diet had less chance of developing breast cancer than women who ate a traditional Western diet.

Crack open a nutty healer

Are you nuts about nuts? If so, you'll like this good news. Adding nuts to a Mediterranean diet — a handful a day for a year — worked even better in one study than adding more olive oil to lower the chances of metabolic syndrome. That's a combination of risk factors for diabetes and heart disease that includes high blood pressure, obesity, and high cholesterol and blood sugar. Add a daily snack of as few as three whole walnuts or seven to eight whole almonds or hazelnuts to get these benefits.

Nuts are chock-full of healthy fats, protein, fiber, and important minerals, like potassium, calcium, and magnesium. They also boast lots of antioxidants. Walnuts and pecans, in particular, have super-high ORAC scores, a measure of antioxidant power.

Here's what nuts can do for your heart.

Bring down high cholesterol. Almonds, macadamia nuts, and pistachios are rich sources of monounsaturated fats. Eating these "good" fats regularly helps lower your "bad" LDL cholesterol. Pistachios also have phytosterols, plant compounds shown to raise your "good" HDL cholesterol. Besides that, eating healthy fats instead of unhealthy saturated fats in meat and butter does your heart a big favor.

Balance your blood sugar. Some nuts, like almonds, help your heart by lowering your body's glycemic response, so your blood sugar doesn't jump sky-high after a meal. Remember that almonds are on the list of six key foods to eat every day as part of the heart-healthy Polymeal.

Tame high blood pressure. Foods with lots of linoleic acid, like sunflower seeds, lower your risk of developing high blood pressure. Research proves it works. In addition, eating more nuts of various kinds lowers your risk of heart disease — but don't overdo these high-calorie treats. Salted varieties have lots of sodium. Keep it to about one-quarter cup a day.

Seafood benefits outweigh risks

The average American eats 16 pounds of seafood every year. Be sure yours is not contaminated. Some fish, especially large predators that eat smaller fish, may contain toxins like mercury and polychlorinated biphenyls (PCBs). Mercury buildup in your body can cause nerve damage or heart problems, while PCBs may cause cancer.

But don't give up eating fish, since the potential benefits outweigh the risks. Just avoid eating swordfish, shark, king mackerel, and tilefish, which are high in mercury. Limit eating tuna steaks, halibut, and red snapper to once a month. Aim for two servings a week of safer options.

- Stick to fish like salmon, flounder, and farm-raised channel catfish and rainbow trout, with low levels of mercury.

- Pick frozen portions typically not made from large predator fish.

- Remove belly and back fat and skin from fish to strip away PCBs.

Angling for a healthy heart

You need to eat some fat, so pick the type that can help your heart. Replace saturated fats from meat with unsaturated fats from fish and plants, and your heart will thank you.

Years of research proves what a miracle food fish can be for your heart. A recent study of middle-age men in Japan and the United States found that those who ate lots of fish had double the blood levels of omega-3 fatty acids. That gave them a lower risk of heart disease. People in Japan tend to eat about 3 ounces of fish every day, while Americans typically eat fish only twice a week.

Those helpful omega-3 fatty acids in oily fish include eicosapentaenoic acid (EPA) and docosahexaenoic acid (DHA). You need these omega-3s, plus the omega-6 fatty acids you'll get from foods like corn oil and sunflower oil and the omega-9 fatty acids in canola oil. All three types of essential fatty acids are important to your body, but people who eat a Western diet get lots more omega-6 fats than omega-3s — a ratio of about 10 to one. Experts say a more balanced mix of the three is healthier.

As you eat more omega-3 fatty acids, your heart will reap these benefits.

- Lower cholesterol and triglycerides.

- Slower buildup of arterial plaque. Omega-3 fatty acids coat your arteries like a nonstick spray, keeping your blood flowing smoothly.

- More flexible arteries to help lower high blood pressure.

- Less chance of heart attack and a lower risk of death from congestive heart failure.

It's easy to add more omega-3 fatty acids to your diet. First, order oily fish — like salmon — instead of steak next time you treat yourself to a meal out. But skip the deep frying and breaded coatings, which add more fat and calories.

When you eat at home, pour on the omega-3s by brushing olive oil on a filet of fish, sprinkling it with Italian spices, then broiling it in the oven on both sides. It's easy, cheap, and combines two great sources of omega-3s. Or look for a new generation of frozen fish that's tastier and healthier than traditional breaded fish sticks. You'll find pan-seared or grilled salmon and sole in the freezer section of your grocery store. But stay away from farm-raised tilapia, since it has high levels of omega-6 fatty acids but not very much omega-3. Farm-raised tilapia is fed corn, high in omega-6 fatty acids, so the fish has as much omega-6 as hamburger or bacon.

You can also take fish oil supplements or eat flaxseed or walnuts to get extra omega-3 fatty acids. Alpha-linolenic acid (ALA) in these plant foods is converted in your body into useful omega-3s. You'll find more and more foods offered with added omega-3s, including eggs, yogurt, and orange juice.

Little-known fish hazard

Eating fatty fish or taking fish oil supplements is a smart idea for most people — but not for everyone. Studies show that people with hard-to-control angina, very poor heart function, or arrhythmias in their lower heart chambers — like ventricular tachycardia — shouldn't eat a lot of fish or take fish oil supplements.

Experts speculate that omega-3 fatty acids work to block certain cells in the heart that typically cause arrhythmias. Usually, that's a good thing. But if your heart is damaged and you don't have enough healthy cells, the omega-3s may keep your heart from having the rhythm it needs to keep going.

Ask your doctor before you try the fish oil treatment if you have an implantable cardioverter defibrillator (ICD), serious angina, or congestive heart failure.

A trans fat that's good for your heart

Trans fats — those troublesome fats found in packaged baked goods, stick margarine, and french fries — can contribute to heart disease by raising your cholesterol level. Some cities, like Boston and New York, have banned them from restaurants. But not all trans fats are bad.

Artificial trans fats, also known as partially hydrogenated oils, are made by adding hydrogen to vegetable oil to create a cheap, solid fat for baking and frying. These fats raise your "bad" LDL cholesterol.

Natural trans fats are different. They're found in meat and dairy products, and they don't raise your cholesterol level. Called trans vaccenic acids, they may actually help by blocking the absorption of harmful fats and cholesterol formed in your intestines from the food you eat.

On the other hand, saturated fats in meat and full-fat dairy products may cause harm, including high cholesterol, high triglycerides, and problems with blood flow to your heart. Pick lean meat and low-fat dairy when you can.

Why you should eat chocolate

Life is good. You can help your heart and eat chocolate, too. That's because dark chocolate fights heart disease, high blood pressure, and other ailments. Here's how it works. Flavonoids and resveratrol, natural plant chemicals in chocolate, behave as antioxidants, fighting free radicals. This prevents damage to cells that can lead to heart disease.

Dark chocolate lowers levels of C-reactive protein, a marker of harmful inflammation in your body. This antioxidant effect also allows chocolate to improve blood vessel function and reduce high blood pressure. In addition, dark chocolate improves your cholesterol profile. In one study, people who ate dark chocolate enjoyed lower "bad" LDL cholesterol and higher "good" HDL cholesterol.

Most people think of grapes when they hear resveratrol. Researchers at the Hershey Company compared levels of resveratrol in various foods and found that cocoa powder, baking chocolate, and dark chocolate are all good sources. These ranked second only to red wine and grape juice.

But never eat your chocolate with a glass of milk. Research shows drinking milk with chocolate reduces the health benefits. That's because milk blocks absorption of antioxidants from the chocolate, so they can't do your body much good. Skip the chocolate milk, and pick dark chocolate over milk chocolate.

Don't overindulge in your favorite chocolate treat, thinking you're helping your heart. Aim for about 7 grams of dark chocolate a day. That's about the size of one and one-half Hershey's Kisses. Beyond that amount, there's no greater benefit, and the excess could add extra pounds to your waistline.

Eat like the French to stay young

Lower cholesterol, stronger blood vessels, less chance of heart disease — even a body that's younger on the inside. Where can you sign up? Turn back the clock for your heart and the rest of your body with these natural plant chemicals in grapes.

Resveratrol. Grapes are a great source of resveratrol, a natural compound that does wonders to keep your heart — and the rest of you — young. Resveratrol encourages the growth of new blood vessels, lowers inflammation, and may even slow aging. It's an antioxidant, so it blocks the harmful free radicals that can damage cells and bring on heart disease and other serious health problems.

Resveratrol, found in the skins of grapes, keeps the fruit healthy by helping the plant fend off stresses like fungus and bad weather. Red wine has more resveratrol than white wine, because the grape skins are left in the wine longer during production. Resveratrol seems to function at the cellular level to slow aging, just like a calorie-restricted diet does. When you get fewer calories than your body thinks it needs, changes take place that slow down the aging process. But you can skip the unhealthy crash diet and enjoy some purple grape juice instead.

This phytochemical in grapes, wine, and grape juice may explain the "French paradox." People in France, who usually drink red wine with meals, seem to be able to eat food high in saturated fat, like butter and cheese, yet have lower rates of heart disease and obesity than Americans.

Pterostilbene. Grapes and blueberries also have pterostilbene, a natural plant compound and antioxidant that can lower your cholesterol better than prescription drugs. It worked wonders on hamsters who had high cholesterol, bringing it down even better than the common cholesterol drug ciprofibrate. Scientists are also studying pterostilbene to see how it can help prevent colon cancer.

Quercetin. Another great phytochemical in grape skins is quercetin, known for its many health benefits. Researchers found a lower risk of heart disease in people who consume more quercetin. This natural plant chemical is also abundant in apples and red onions.

You can get the benefits of these powerful phytochemicals from grapes, grape juice, or wine. Pick purple grape juice rather than white, and look for one made of real fruit juice with little or no sugar added.

If you enjoy an occasional drink, stick to wine rather than other forms of alcohol. Many researchers think it's not the alcohol in wine that's helpful but the natural plant chemicals. In fact, alcohol can cause other problems for your heart, like raise your blood pressure or worsen an irregular heartbeat, and some people can become alcohol dependent.

Supplements are available, including some that contain both resveratrol and quercetin. Look for a brand called Resvinatrol Complete, which has quercetin and more resveratrol than a large bottle of grape juice or red wine.

Grounds for concern

Don't drink coffee too close to your daily trip to the gym if you have heart disease. Wait at least five hours after you sip a cup before you exercise. Experts think the caffeine in coffee limits your body's ability to increase blood flow to your heart during aerobic activity.

People with healthy hearts can handle the change, but if you have heart disease, your heart has to work extra hard to pump blood through narrowed arteries. Play it safe and don't drink more than two cups of regular coffee a day if you have heart disease.

Win half the day's nutritional battle with breakfast

Start your day with a heart-healthy breakfast to keep your arteries clear, your cholesterol down, and heart disease at bay. Statistics prove it. You're most at risk of cardiac arrest first thing in the morning. That's because your body is low in fluids after a night spent sleeping — not eating and drinking. In addition, studies show people who eat breakfast tend to have lower cholesterol than people who skip it. So refuel first thing. Here's what's on your best-bet menu.

Oatmeal. Enjoying a bowl of oatmeal is one easy thing you can do every day to lower your cholesterol. It's much simpler than taking drugs or seeing a doctor. The soluble fiber in oats brings down the "bad" LDL cholesterol in your blood without changing your "good" HDL cholesterol. Benefits to your heart are so powerful oatmeal makers are allowed to include this claim right on the label. Go for plain oatmeal rather than sugar-sweetened packets of instant oatmeal.

Whole-grain toast with the right spread. Check the label on your bread to be sure it's 100-percent whole grain. Something called "wheat" bread just won't do — it's still refined grain. You need the entire grain seed — bran, germ, and endosperm — to get all the fiber, vitamins, minerals, and healthy fats that help your heart. In fact, studies show that people who eat at least two-and-a-half servings of whole grains every day can lower their risk of heart disease by 21 percent.

Stay away from the artery-clogging saturated fat in butter. Instead, use a spread that contains phytosterols, plant substances that block cholesterol absorption in your intestines. Called stanols or sterols, they can help lower your cholesterol. Look for brands like Benecol and Promise Activ margarine. You need two to three tablespoons a day for the most benefits.

Orange juice or a whole orange. One extra serving a day of this mouthwatering fruit can reduce your risk of stroke, lower obesity, and fight heart disease. No wonder it's a morning favorite.

The hefty serving of vitamin C you get from an orange or a glass of orange juice — along with more than 170 different phytochemicals — give this treat its antioxidant and other disease-fighting powers. Folate in orange juice lowers your stroke risk.

Researchers also found that people who drank three cups of OJ every day lowered their LDL-HDL cholesterol ratio by 16 percent and raised their HDL by 21 percent. This keeps your arteries unclogged and crystal clear.

Enjoy the perks of a cuppa 'joe'

Make a daily cup of coffee part of your morning routine, and you'll do more than feel awake and alert. You'll also be doing your heart good. One study found that coffee drinkers tend to live longer, and it's because they have a lower risk of dying of heart-related problems like heart attack and stroke.

The caffeine in coffee is not what saves lives, since decaf drinkers had similar protection. Instead, scientists think it's the antioxidant phenols in coffee beans that help. In addition, acids in coffee — caffeic, ferulic, and p-coumaric acids — keep low-density lipoproteins, or LDL cholesterol, from oxidizing and causing inflammation.

Researchers at Harvard Medical School found that women who drank five to seven cups of coffee a week were less likely to have a stroke than those who drank it only once a month. Stroke protection likely comes from coffee's antioxidants, which reduce inflammation and protect your blood vessels.

But drinking coffee isn't a good idea for everyone. Follow this advice from health professionals.

- Avoid unfiltered varieties like Turkish or French press coffee. These unfiltered types have more cafestol, a natural compound that can raise your LDL cholesterol levels. Stick to filtered coffee.

- Some people carry a gene that causes slower breakdown of caffeine, putting them at higher risk of coffee-related heart attacks. So far there's no test to see if you're one of those folks.

- If you have heart disease and are not a regular coffee drinker, a splurge could increase your risk of suffering a heart attack or stroke.

- Don't drink regular coffee if you have high blood pressure, since the caffeine can worsen your condition.

Sip your way to good health

Lower your blood pressure and help your heart with delicious green tea. You'll improve your health while you enjoy your fill of this soothing, refreshing drink considered a healing beverage since the time of the ancient Chinese.

Some of that is due to powerful antioxidants called catechins. You've probably heard of an important catechin, epigallocatechin-3-gallate (EGCG). Green tea has more antioxidant power than black tea — even more than vegetables like brussels sprouts or spinach. It also has certain vitamins and minerals that help these antioxidants perform better.

Nutrients in green tea help your heart and keep your arteries flexible. In fact, numerous studies show drinking green tea regularly may lower your blood pressure, prevent heart disease, and improve the health of your arteries. But it's important to pick green tea over its black cousin. Some experts say drinking black tea may actually raise your blood pressure, possibly because of its caffeine.

Get into the habit of drinking green tea, and you'll keep the rest of your body in tiptop shape. Here's what the nutrients in green tea can do for you.

- Keep your bones strong. Some studies show green tea improves bone density and prevents hip fracture.

- Keep your brain sharp. Experts think the polyphenols — natural plant compounds — in green tea may protect against Parkinson's disease and Alzheimer's disease.

- Keep your belly lean. Some people believe the catechins in green tea make your body burn fat faster. Give it a try.

Add a splash of orange, lemon, or lime juice to your tea to boost these benefits. A couple tablespoons of citrus juice in a cup makes the catechins more stable, so they can get to your body and do some good. For the highest level of catechins, brew regular green tea fresh. Instant, iced, and decaffeinated green tea have fewer catechins.

For most people, there's no limit to how much green tea you can drink. But if you're taking a statin drug, don't overindulge in green tea. Too much — three or more cups a day — seems to cause statins to build up in your blood, possibly causing muscle pain. Drink less green tea to avoid this potential interaction.

Short-circuit high blood pressure with herbal tea

Herbal tea may help lower your blood pressure, so give it a try if you don't like green tea. Investigators found that people with high blood pressure who drank three or more cups of herbal tea with hibiscus every day had great results in just six weeks.

Their blood pressure was lower by an average of 7 points systolic, the first number in a blood pressure reading. Tea worked best for people who had the highest blood pressure. Most herbal tea blends sold in the United States contain hibiscus.

4 must-have pantry items for better health

Together they protect you against almost all diseases of aging — plus they make your food taste better. Put these four must-have items in your spice rack or pantry, and your heart will say, "Mm, mm, good."

Cinnamon. You don't need to have high blood pressure when cinnamon can keep it under control. Animal studies show cinnamon lowers your blood pressure. Merely smelling the cinnamon from an apple pie makes you feel calm and relaxed. Eating it does even more.

Cinnamon's effect on blood pressure seems to be related to the spice's ability to lower levels of insulin in your body. The right balance of blood sugar and insulin helps keep blood pressure stable. Besides that, taking only one-half teaspoon of cinnamon powder twice daily before a meal can keep your blood sugar under control and lower your cholesterol.

Garlic. Learn to love the taste and smell of this lifesaving herb. Natural compounds, like allicin and selenium, mean garlic can inhibit cancer growth, prevent blood clots, and lower cholesterol. Garlic may even bring down your blood pressure. Allicin works like an ACE-inhibiting drug and helps your blood vessels expand to keep blood flowing smoothly.

That's a lot of good health — just from enjoying a delicious herb. For the most powerful benefits for your heart, choose fresh garlic. But if you truly can't take the heat of this pungent herb, try garlic supplements.

Ginger. You know this soothing spice for the way it relieves nausea. Ginger is also a boon for your heart. A study in Iran found that people who ate ginger three times a day for 45 days had lower LDL — the "bad" kind of cholesterol. Active compounds called gingerols give this ancient spice its healing powers.

Turmeric. People in ancient India relied on curcumin, turmeric's active ingredient, to treat skin diseases, digestive problems, inflammatory joint disorders, and a variety of infections. Modern research shows curcumin works as an antioxidant and anti-inflammatory to battle the chronic inflammation that's linked to heart disease. Research shows it may fend off heart enlargement and heart failure. This spice may also fight tumors in your colon and pancreas.

Shake the salt habit to live longer

Cutting salt intake in half would prevent 150,000 deaths in America every year. That's a lot of lives saved with just a little change. Find out where most of your salt comes from and how you can start cutting back without losing flavor.

The problem with salt is it's half sodium. Getting too much sodium can lead to high blood pressure, kidney damage, heart disease, and stroke. Sodium in your body causes your kidneys to release more fluid, adding volume to your blood. That raises blood pressure and puts stress on your blood vessels. If your blood pressure is consistently at or above 140/90 mmHg, you have hypertension, or high blood pressure.

Keep a lid on it. Healthy people should limit sodium intake to no more than 2,300 milligrams (mg) a day, or about a teaspoon of table salt. But people with high blood pressure and people middle-age or older should limit it to 1,500 mg of sodium. A typical American eats about 3,400 mg of sodium every day, and most of it isn't from a salt shaker. About three-fourths comes from processed foods, like frozen dinners, canned food, and meals in restaurants.

Toss your shaker. Skip the salt and replace it with this lifesaving substitute. A potassium-enriched salt substitute, like Morton Lite Salt or Cardia Salt, balances the sodium and potassium in your body. These two minerals work together to regulate fluids. Boosting your potassium intake can help lower your blood pressure.

You can also find salt-free seasonings, like Mrs. Dash or Spike, that add flavor to your food without increasing the sodium content. Experts are also working on other kinds of low-sodium salt alternatives, like Seagreens seaweed granules, which contain other important minerals.

Help your heart. High blood pressure is a major risk factor for heart-related illness. A better balance of minerals could reduce deaths from heart disease, diabetes, high blood pressure, and stroke. Researchers found that veterans who switched to a potassium-enriched salt lived longer and had less heart-related illness than those who didn't switch.

If you're on a low-salt or low-potassium diet or take a potassium-sparing diuretic, ask your doctor before you try one of these products.

Apricots score an A+ for smart snacking

Why not enjoy apricots — the fruit people eat to avoid cancer, heart disease, and Alzheimer's disease. These tasty gems are loaded with powerful weapons that could even help you live longer. Here are six ways apricots promote good health.

Rescue your heart. The potassium in apricots — 40 percent of your daily requirement in a cup of dried fruit — helps to regulate your blood pressure, avoid heart disease, and sidestep high cholesterol. This important mineral weakens the effect of sodium in your body. It works so well that some experts think a potassium-rich diet may cut your risk of stroke by up to 40 percent. Soluble fiber in apricots also keeps your blood pressure low, while it brings down your cholesterol.

Sidestep cancer. Lycopene, the carotenoid that makes tomatoes red and apricots orange, may cut men's risk of prostate cancer. The body stores some lycopene in the prostate.

Avoid Alzheimer's disease. Experts think fruits with lots of antioxidant power, including apricots and blueberries, may help you steer clear of the mind-stealing effects of Alzheimer's disease.

Fight fatigue. Too little iron in your blood can make you anemic. But even people who don't have anemia may benefit from iron, feeling more energetic and less fatigued. Get that iron from apricots. A cup of dried apricots has nearly 20 percent of the iron you need in a day.

Improve your skin, hair, and nails. Iron in your diet can also help keep your hair healthy — and on your head. In fact, iron supplements are sometimes given to battle hair loss. Eat apricots to get more iron naturally. Besides that, the hefty helping of vitamin A in apricots helps keep your skin and nails healthy and strong.

Keep digestion moving smoothly. Apricots have both soluble and insoluble fiber, with a total of more than 3 grams in a cup of dried fruit. That makes them your digestive system's best friend. Enjoy them fresh or dried — only 16 calories each.

Modern benefits from an ancient treat

Got a sweet tooth? Try charoset, a delicious dessert as old as the hills. At Passover, many Jews enjoy this mixture of fruit, nuts, wine, cinnamon, and honey. It forms a delicious, thick paste symbolizing the mortar their enslaved Hebrew ancestors used to build the cities of Egypt. This delicious dessert contains ingredients known to fight cancer, reduce heart attack risk, ease angina pain, lower blood sugar, and cure infections.

Apples. This super fruit can ease arthritis, raise good cholesterol levels, boost lung power, and aid digestion. Apples also may help prevent lung cancer and protect you from heart disease. The generous amounts of fiber, minerals like boron, and natural plant chemicals called phytochemicals in apples make them a nutritional powerhouse.

Bananas. Enjoy this great source of potassium to balance out too much sodium in your diet. Bananas also keep high cholesterol in check and prevent bad LDL cholesterol from oxidizing and harming your arteries.

Cinnamon. This fragrant spice lowers blood pressure, fights infection, and keeps your blood sugar stable. The antioxidant power of cinnamon may get full credit for these benefits.

Walnuts. These little nutritional nuggets are rich in omega-3 fatty acids, which reduce inflammation and prevent blood clots. Their heart-healthy fats may also give your HDL cholesterol a boost.

To make charoset, peel and grate one-half cup of cooking apples and set aside. Use a food processor to finely chop one-half cup of walnuts. Add a handful of dates, three bananas, two tablespoons of honey, two teaspoons of cinnamon, and one-fourth cup of sweet red wine. Blend until smooth. Pour the blended mixture over the grated apples and mix well. The charoset should have the consistency of wet cement. Spread on crackers and enjoy.

'Value' vanilla poses heart risk

Cheap imitation vanilla extract from Mexico tempts your wallet, but the savings are risky. Some imitation vanilla extract is made from tonka beans, not real vanilla beans or acceptable imitation flavorings. Tonka beans contain coumarin, a toxic substance banned from food in the United States. Coumarin is related to warfarin (Coumadin), a blood-thinning drug. It may be risky to eat coumarin if you're taking a blood thinner. The interaction can increase bleeding.

Sidestep the risk by avoiding cheap vanilla if you're traveling in Mexico or other Latin American countries. Also, be wary of vanilla you buy in the United States that's not labeled in English or that doesn't say "vanilla bean" on the label.

Meet the king of the berries

Skip the pale juices. Pick juice in more exciting colors of red, purple, and blue. Those darker hues are signs of good nutrition. Berries like blueberries, cranberries, and açai all contain powerful antioxidants that give them their dark colors. Research shows blueberries can lower cholesterol, thus keeping your arteries clear and reducing your risk of heart disease. Other studies show cranberry juice may lower your cholesterol.

But the small purple açai berry is king of the dark berries, with its high ORAC (oxygen radical absorbance capacity) score, a measure of antioxidant power. Get a leg up on the fight against aging, heart disease, cancer, and Alzheimer's disease with açai juice — a delicious juice made from the world's highest antioxidant fruit. High ORAC scores mean the fruit has a powerful ability to neutralize free radicals in your body. If these unstable molecules were left to roam free, they would harm cells, potentially allowing cancer, heart disease, and Alzheimer's disease to progress.

Açai — pronounced ah-sigh-EE — earns its "super fruit" reputation with an ORAC of 102,700 for freeze-dried berries. It's from the Amazonian palm tree in South America, the same tree that hearts of palm come from. Açai is also high in potassium, fiber, B vitamins, and omega-3 fatty acids, so it's an all-around winner for your heart. Berries from closer to home that also boast great ORAC scores include cranberries at ORAC 9,584 and blueberries at 6,552. Be aware that only the purple açai — not the white variety — has this high antioxidant capacity.

Açai is not always easy to find, plus it's expensive. Use a little açai juice and blend it into a treat with all three fabulous berries — açai, blueberries, and cranberries. Check the labels to be sure you're buying real fruit juice, not "cocktails" with little juice and lots of sugar. If you have to resort to mail order to buy açai, know that some companies don't produce the quality of juice they claim and may have questionable billing practices.

Unexpected source of powerful antioxidants

Prefer veggies to fruits? You'll also get a heapin' helpin' of antioxidants from beans — the darker the better.

"Black beans are really loaded with antioxidant compounds," says researcher Clifford Beninger. "We didn't know they were that potent until now. It's maybe a bit of a wake-up call that we should be eating more beans."

Beninger and colleagues tested 12 common beans to see which have the most antioxidant flavonoids, pigments found in their skin. It seems darker is better when it comes to beans, just like with fruit. Black beans beat out red, brown, yellow, and white beans, in that order.

Tricks to tame dangerous acrylamides

Go easy on potato chips and french fries — and other foods that contain lots of acrylamides. That's the latest advice from the U.S. Food and Drug Administration (FDA). Acrylamides were already suspected to cause cancer and damage your nervous system. Now researchers think they can harm your heart, too.

Acrylamides are harmful compounds that can form in carbohydrate-rich foods cooked at high heat — frying, roasting, or baking. That includes potato chips, french fries, and some cereals and roasted coffees. Studies show eating too much food with high acrylamide content brings on your body's inflammatory response and raises levels of C-reactive proteins. That increases the oxidative stress on your body, and it can make heart disease worse.

Experts admit that the participants in one study ate about three times as much acrylamides as you'll find in a typical Western diet. They ate 160 grams of potato chips — or about the same amount as four snack-size bags — every day for 28 days. Although the researchers needed to study impact in short-term, they suspect long-term exposure to high levels of acrylamide-containing foods would have a similar effect — inflammation and heart disease.

You can reduce your acrylamide intake by cutting down on foods like potato chips and french fries. Try these tricks to cut acry-lamides that form in cooking.

- Bake or boil potatoes rather than frying.

- Slice up potatoes and soak them in cold water for two hours before cooking. This will cut the acrylamide content by nearly half. If you really want french fries, fry them in virgin olive oil.

- Mix fresh rosemary into bread dough before baking.

An eating plan that's easy to love

Instead of "eat your vegetables," the best advice may be to "eat only your vegetables" — plus some fruit, low-fat milk, eggs, and whole grains. Your heart will sing the praises of a vegetarian eating plan.

Skipping meat may also help your waistline. People who followed a meatless diet lost more weight than those on a standard low-fat diet, and they had more success sticking to the plan. The meatless plan was an ovo-lacto vegetarian diet, which includes eggs and dairy products but no red meat, poultry, or fish. Those who ate meatless lost more than 16 pounds in a year, eating fewer calories and less fat. They also saw their "bad" LDL cholesterol go down during that time. Even better, they liked this low-cholesterol diet so much they were able to stay on it — even after they lost the extra weight.

You may not consider yourself a vegetarian, but giving up meat may be easier than you think. What's more, you'll get to know a variety of tasty vegetables and grains. It's also healthier than you can imagine. The saturated fat in meat can raise your cholesterol. And people who eat lots of red and processed meat are more likely to die of cancer or heart disease. Get help finding vegetarian foods you like at *www.vrg.org*, the Web site of The Vegetarian Resource Group. All elements of the meatless diet help your heart.

Leafy greens. People who eat more green leafy vegetables, like spinach, kale, and romaine lettuce, have fewer problems with arrhythmia, or an irregular heartbeat, and heart disease. It's best to steam your greens, broccoli, and bell peppers to improve their health benefits. This kind of cooking allows the veggies to bind bile acids, keeping your body from absorbing lots of fat from food. That boosts heart benefits.

Dairy. Drinking milk, especially low-fat or fat-free milk, may improve your blood protein profile. That's a sign of good kidney function and less risk of heart disease. Milk may also lower your blood pressure and cut your risk of metabolic syndrome, a combination of risk factors for diabetes and heart disease that includes high blood pressure, obesity, and high cholesterol and blood sugar.

Vitamin D in milk may lower your risk of heart attack and other heart-related problems. For detailed information on taking vitamin D as a supplement or getting this nutrient from sunshine, go to "Beat disease with the sunshine vitamin" on page 82 in *Cardio health: fit for life*.

Eggs. Think eggs are forbidden if you have high cholesterol? Think again. It's true egg yolks contain a good bit of dietary cholesterol, but dietary cholesterol is only one factor that affects your body's cholesterol level. Others include smoking, being overweight, and not exercising. Experts say eating eggs regularly won't raise your blood cholesterol. In fact, an egg a day has been shown to improve your balance of HDL and LDL cholesterol. Keep in mind other studies have hinted at health risks from eating more than six eggs a week, especially if you have diabetes.

Egg protein is a complete protein, which is important if you're not eating meat. In fact, some experts say certain proteins in eggs actually function like ACE-inhibitor drugs in your body, bringing down high blood pressure.

Whole grains. Don't forget this important component of your ovo-lacto vegetarian diet. Some studies show people who eat at least a couple servings every day of whole grains — like whole-wheat bread, brown rice, or oatmeal — have a lower risk of heart disease and stroke.

Remarkable mushroom boosts vitamin D

Food experts are working hard to help you get the vitamin D you need. The U.S. Department of Agriculture helped develop new Monterey Sun-Bella mushrooms to make that easier.

Sun-Bella mushrooms are regular mushrooms that were exposed to sunlight while they were growing, so they've captured lots of the sunshine vitamin. Each 3-ounce serving gives you a full day's requirement of vitamin D. Mushrooms don't have fat or cholesterol, so they're naturally good for your heart. Look for Sun-Bella mushrooms at your favorite grocers, including Albertsons, Kroger, and Whole Foods.

3 little-known reasons to eat flaxseed

Don't be flummoxed about flaxseed. It's not a health food store rarity anymore. And this tiny seed has three great things going for it — fiber, alpha-linolenic acid, and lignans.

Fiber. Flaxseed is nearly one-third fiber, both soluble and insoluble. That may be why you can sweep artery-clogging cholesterol right out of your system with this little seed. Studies show people who ate a few tablespoons of ground flaxseed every day for just four weeks lowered their total cholesterol and "bad" LDL cholesterol, but the "good" HDL cholesterol stayed the same.

There are so many good ingredients in flaxseed, experts have trouble telling what it is that has this cholesterol-lowering effect. They think it could be both the mucilage gums, a soluble fiber in flaxseed, and alpha-linolenic acid (ALA), an important omega-3 fatty acid that helps your heart. Flaxseed is the richest plant source of ALA.

Alpha-linolenic acid. One study found that men with the highest levels of ALA stored in their body fat had the lowest risk of a heart attack. Experts say the protection came from eating as little as one-half teaspoon of flaxseed oil daily. ALA works by blocking chronic inflammation in your body, which over time can lead to heart attack and stroke.

Lignans. Flaxseed is also a great source of lignans, natural plant hormones. These estrogen-like compounds are in the shell of flaxseed, not in the oil. They can lower your cholesterol to reduce your risk of heart disease and stroke. Lignans may also safely ease your menopause symptoms and protect against cancers of the breast, colon, and prostate.

Flaxseed has a pleasant, nutty taste, so you'll enjoy this healthy addition to many foods. Aim for one to two tablespoons of ground flaxseed or one to two teaspoons of flaxseed oil to get these health benefits. You'll find flaxseed added to a number of tasty foods like these.

- baked goods, like bagels, muffins, and multigrain bread

- packaged cereal, pasta, and pancake mix

- ice cream and other frozen treats

Or buy whole or ground flaxseed and flaxseed oil, and use them in your own cooking and baking. Look for them in your health food store or local grocery.

Discover the power of lupin flour

Next time you get a taste for something new, heed the call of the wild. Wild flowers, that is. Seeds of the lupin plant — a family of beautiful wildflowers that includes the Texas bluebonnet — make great-tasting and good-for-you foods.

Lupin flowers grow in long stalks of a dozen small buds, often purple. The plant's kernels are milled to make a pale yellow flour, popular in Europe and Australia. Lupin kernel flour is a health nut's dream, with up to 45 percent protein and 30 percent fiber, but little sugar or starch. Research shows its many health benefits.

Lowers blood pressure. Overweight people who ate lupin flour bread for four months lowered their blood pressure by 3 mmHg systolic, the first number in a blood pressure reading. The special bread was made by substituting lupin flour for 40 percent of the wheat flour. Lupin flour has several ingredients that could get credit, including a high level of arginine, an amino acid your body needs to make nitric oxide. This gas relaxes blood vessels to lower blood pressure.

Reduces cholesterol levels. Men who ate foods containing lupin fiber for a month had lower total cholesterol and "bad" LDL cholesterol. Experts think the high fiber content of lupin was the reason.

Quiets your appetite. People who ate lupin bread for breakfast felt fuller than those who ate white bread. They stayed full and ate less at lunch.

Food manufacturers are adding lupin flour to pasta, cakes, cookies, bread, and chips. Look for these items, along with lupin flour for baking, in health food stores and the gourmet section of your supermarket. But if you're allergic to peanuts or other foods, be careful about trying lupin. You may also be allergic to this plant.

Sour news on sweet drinks

Want one easy change you can make in your diet that will really benefit your heart? Cut out the sugary drinks. Research shows that women who regularly drink sweetened beverages — both sodas and noncarbonated drinks — have a higher risk of heart disease. These results held true even when researchers accounted for other risk factors, like being overweight and having diabetes.

Experts point out that drinking a sweetened beverage increases your blood sugar and insulin levels, leading to a rise in C-reactive protein — a marker of inflammation. Lowering your level of C-reactive protein is just as important as lowering your cholesterol to reduce your heart attack risk.

Heal your arteries with tomatoes

The American Heart Association's "Go Red for Women" campaign reminds women they're not immune to heart disease. Take that cue, and add ruby-red tomatoes to your plate whenever you can. You'll dance your way through your golden years.

You don't have to suffer a heart attack if you make "love apples" a regular part of your diet. Eat them in a salad, simmered into a tasty pasta sauce, as a bowl of tomato soup, or in a glass of tomato juice. This garden treat is a great source of the nutrient lycopene — a carotenoid known for its role in preventing prostate cancer — and it's what makes tomatoes red. But lycopene also does several things to reduce your heart disease risk.

- Lowers LDL cholesterol. Lycopene worked better than a statin drug in one study to lower cholesterol.

- Works as an antioxidant. Research in middle-age men with heart disease found that antioxidants protect your arteries from damage caused by unstable molecules called free radicals.

- Stops blood clots. Drinking tomato extract blocks the formation of blood clots, which can trigger a heart attack.

- Reduces blood pressure. People with high blood pressure who drank tomato extract for eight weeks lowered their systolic and diastolic blood pressure.

You get the largest portion of lycopene from tomato products, like tomato juice and tomato sauce, but slicing a few tomatoes onto your salad is a start at incorporating these tasty summer treats into your diet. If you don't relish tomatoes, scientists recently developed a "tomato pill," or lycopene supplement, called Ateronon.

Dress your salad well or add the right ingredient to your tomato sauce, and tomatoes become even healthier. If you put a little oil on your salad, it will draw more heart-saving antioxidants from your veggies. Research shows carotenoids are better absorbed by your body from veggies in a salad with full-fat dressing rather than low-fat or fat-free dressing.

To do your heart the most good, pick a salad dressing made with olive oil, make an olive oil and vinegar dressing, or add avocados for an interesting source of healthy fat. If you're cooking down tomatoes into marinara sauce, add a tad of olive oil. Your taste buds will be delighted.

Go green for your heart's sake

Your mom was right. Eating your vegetables will keep you healthy. It's easy eating green — from the exotic to the everyday.

Broccoli. This traditional favorite works to prevent cancer, plus it's great for your heart. Research in lab rats found eating broccoli helped them produce more heart-protecting protein called thioredoxin. That helps your heart pump better, so there's less damage during a heart attack.

Like other cruciferous vegetables, including cauliflower and cabbage, broccoli is high in the phytochemical sulforaphane. This antioxidant works to prevent blood vessel damage from high blood sugar in diabetes. Sulforaphane boosts your body's immune system to help you age gracefully — and healthfully. You'll also get the nutrient choline from broccoli. Choline is related to the B vitamins, and it's important for healthy nerves. It also helps lower C-reactive protein — a sign of inflammation and damaged arteries.

Dark leafy greens. Kale and spinach are fabulous sources of vitamin K. This vitamin, named "K" for "koagulation" by a Danish scientist, helps your blood clot.

Your heart benefits from vitamin K. It can block chronic inflammation and slow down hardening of the arteries. A study in middle-age women found that those who got more vitamin K in their diets had less thickening of the aorta. That's important to let blood flow freely from your heart.

But vitamin K can interfere with blood-thinning drugs like warfarin (Coumadin), so talk to your doctor before you make a change in your diet if you're taking a blood thinner.

Seaweed. Get to know seaweed, the vegetable that's been popular in Asian countries for centuries. This low-calorie, fat-free vegetable is a better source of minerals than all the other veggies. Plus, it's an anti-inflammatory and stress-reliever, and it can lower your risk of heart disease — a real super food. All three basic types of edible seaweed — green, brown, and red — are common in Asian cuisine. If you like sushi rolls, you're familiar with nori, the kind used as a wrapper.

Certain kinds of seaweed, or sea vegetables, have more calcium than whole milk, more potassium than a banana, and more magnesium and iron than spinach. Some types have more soluble and insoluble fiber than many land-growing plants. Seaweed also can boast of the antioxidant vitamins A, C, and E. It's one of the few vegetable sources of vitamin B12.

These nutrients are great for your heart. The omega-3 fatty acids in seaweed could lower your body's level of C-reactive protein, a major marker of inflammation and heart disease. Finally, eating seaweed may help you bypass the blues. Research found that women who eat more omega-3 fatty acids have fewer symptoms of depression.

Beginner's guide to sea vegetables

You'll find edible seaweed, also called sea vegetables, in Asian food stores, health food stores, or through online grocers, like *www.amazon.com* and *www.netgrocer.com*. It is usually dried soon after it's gathered to preserve freshness. Store it in an airtight opaque container below 70 degrees Fahrenheit. Don't put it in the refrigerator, since it absorbs odors easily.

	How it's sold	Common uses
nori	packaged in square sheets; processed with rice into crackers	roast or fry small pieces; use as wrapper for sushi
sea lettuce	dried and packaged	add to salad and soups; eat out of bag as crunchy snack
dulse	dried and packaged	soak and add to salad, stir-fry dish, or soup
hijiki	dried and packaged	eat out of the bag as crunchy snack
wakame/kombu	dried and packaged; dried and packaged as instant seaweed soup	soak and add to salad, stir-fry dish, or miso soup; brew into a tea

4 ways to strike back at stroke

More than 5 million people die worldwide every year from stroke. But you don't have to be a stroke victim. A simple combination of vitamins, minerals, and other nutrients does the trick. Consider making this quartet of dietary changes.

Stop deadly clots with vitamin C. Pick your favorite vitamin C-packed fruit, like oranges and grapefruit, and you may prevent clogged arteries. This vitamin strengthens your blood vessel walls, which promotes good circulation. Some studies also show vitamin C can prevent blood vessels from constricting and cutting off blood flow to your heart and brain. One study found that people middle-age and older who had the highest levels of vitamin C in their blood had the lowest risk of a stroke over the next decade.

Vitamin C does so much more for you, maybe even saving your eyesight. Researchers in Japan discovered that people who take in the most vitamin C have the lowest risk of cataracts. It could be the result of powerful antioxidants at work.

Oranges are great sources of vitamin C, but if you want something more exotic, try papayas. A single cup of papaya cubes has a full day's supply of vitamin C. This tropical favorite is also high in fiber, vitamin A, potassium, folate, and magnesium. Fiber, magnesium, and potassium benefit your heart by lowering your blood pressure.

Catch fishy protection with essential fatty acids. Reduce your risk of stroke and slash your risk of Alzheimer's at the same time by eating essential fatty acids in fish. People who eat three servings a week of fish — especially tuna or other types high in omega-3 fatty acids — have fewer brain lesions that predict stroke and dementia. You can benefit by eating fish as little as once a week. These healthy fats work like natural aspirin to cut inflammation throughout your body and lower your risk of heart disease, stroke, and dementia.

Pick coffee, tea, or milk. The next time you're looking for something to quench your thirst, keep your heart in mind. All three of these popular beverages can help keep your heart healthy.

- Milk. The hefty serving of calcium in moo-juice also cuts your risk of stroke. The benefit may be due to calcium's ability to lower blood pressure.

- Coffee. Women in the Nurses' Health Study who drank four or more cups of coffee a day lowered their risk of stroke by 20 percent.

- Tea. Whether you like green or black tea, drink at least three cups every day to cut your chances of stroke by 21 percent.

Researchers say the caffeine in coffee and tea is not what protects your heart, so decaf varieties may also help. Tea contains the antioxidant EGCG and the amino acid theanine, while coffee has antioxidant phenols.

Trade refined for whole grains. Eat at least two and one-half servings of whole grains every day, and you'll cut your risk of heart disease and stroke by 21 percent. The bran and germ in whole grains is where you'll find the vitamins, minerals, healthy fats, fiber, and antioxidants. That's why whole-grain breads and cereals beat out products made with refined, white flour.

If people who eat lots of insoluble fiber, like in whole grains, have a stroke, they are able to recover better afterward. Their strokes also tend to be less severe.

Foolproof plan to eat more veggies

A glass of vegetable juice is a tasty option when you crave a refreshing drink. Lots of flavors of vegetable juice are available, from traditional V8 to newer veggie-fruit juice blends. People who drink vegetable juice every day do a good job of getting the recommended amount of vegetables. Plus, they find out they really like it.

Here are the benefits. One study found that men who drank about two-thirds cup of kale juice every day had lower cholesterol levels after just three months. Another study showed beet juice is a good choice. The study participants had lower blood pressure after drinking two cups of beet juice. Even refreshing fruit juices can do your heart good. Pomegranate juice is a winner for lowering blood pressure, reducing inflammation, and keeping your arteries clear. So raise a juice glass to your heart — and make it 100 percent juice without sugar or other additives.

Other natural remedies

Bust vitamin myths wide open

Taking megadoses of vitamins and relying on a multivitamin won't guarantee a healthy heart. But certain vitamins in the right doses are necessary for good heart health. Uncover the latest research to bust these common myths.

Myth #1 — Pop a vitamin pill to prevent disease. People take multivitamins as a kind of insurance — they want to be sure they make up for nutrients they may not be getting from food. But that strategy doesn't always work. The Women's Health Initiative study found that older women who took multivitamins for eight years had no less risk of heart disease, various types of cancers, or dying of any cause than women who didn't take the vitamins.

Myth #2 — Supplements can replace a healthy diet. Even powerhouse antioxidant vitamin supplements don't really protect your heart, although eating a diet with lots of antioxidant-rich fruits and vegetables gives you protection.

The Women's Antioxidant Cardiovascular Study followed middle-age women for more than nine years. Some took supplements of vitamin C, vitamin E, or beta carotene every day, and some didn't. By the end of the study, the women who took supplements were no less likely to have had a stroke, heart attack, heart bypass procedure, or heart-related death than those who didn't take them. Don't waste your money on these vitamins.

Why don't vitamins help? Research showing how certain vitamins work in the lab doesn't always translate to your body. Scientists can't really do a test to remove all the vitamin C from your diet because it's in your diet naturally.

Myth #3 — More is better. Another problem is you can overdo vitamin pills as opposed to getting nutrients from food. Most antioxidants are also pro-oxidants, so they work differently in your body in different situations. When taken in large quantities, they can cause health problems.

For example, a study on vitamins C and E found they may block your body's natural response to exercise. Normally, exercise "teaches" your body to use glucose more efficiently and improves your glucose sensitivity. When the men in the study took these two antioxidant supplements, exercise did not improve their glucose metabolism.

Seek out those top-notch vitamins that really do help your heart, including vitamin D and some B vitamins. Read on for details about how these vitamins keep you healthy.

Beat disease with the sunshine vitamin

"As a general rule, old people need more than young people, big people need more than little people, heavier people need more than skinny people, northern people need more than southern people, dark-skinned people need more than fair-skinned people, winter people need more than summer people, sunblock lovers need more than sunblock haters, sun-phobes need more than sun worshipers, and ill people may need more than well people."

This statement from the Vitamin D Council shows how complicated the issue of vitamin D intake is. But you can't ignore it — this one vitamin is clearly associated with longer life. Yet, even scientists don't know exactly why it works.

Vitamin D is important to keep your bones and muscles healthy and ward off heart disease and some cancers. In fact, a study shows that people with less vitamin D in their blood are twice as likely to die of any cause within the next eight years, although deaths related to heart disease were significant.

You'll find vitamin D in several foods, including oily fish like salmon and tuna, as well as fortified milk. But most people don't get enough in their diets. Sunlight is a major source. Ultraviolet light from the sun reacts with a compound in your skin to produce vitamin D. A light-skinned person needs around 15 minutes in the sun without sunscreen a few times a week to get enough vitamin D from sunlight. Dark-skinned people may need up to six times as much UV exposure. Of course, seasonal differences in the sun affect how much exposure you really need.

Older people have a special problem with lack of vitamin D, often because they don't spend enough time in sunlight. It's especially a problem for house-bound seniors and those who live in nursing homes. Also, older people simply don't process vitamin D from the sun as efficiently as younger people. Experts estimate that 40 to 90 percent of seniors don't get enough of the vitamin for best health.

Vitamin D supplements can ensure you get enough. Current U.S. guidelines call for 400 international units (IU) for people age 51 through 70, and 600 IU after age 70. Other health professionals disagree and say you need more. In fact, one study of women and heart health found that those taking just 400 IU of vitamin D every day had no benefits from the supplements. Experts at the Linus Pauling Institute suggest you get 1,000 to 2,000 IU every day.

There are two types of vitamin D supplements — vitamin D2 (ergocalciferol) and vitamin D3 (cholecalciferol). Vitamin D3 is the form that's most useful for your body. When buying supplements, look for vitamin D3 on the label. Check with your doctor before you take vitamin D supplements if you take calcium-channel blockers or thiazide diuretics.

Too much vitamin D can lead to excess calcium in your blood, causing calcium deposits in your blood vessels, heart, lungs, and kidneys. That can result in kidney damage and even kidney failure.

It's a good idea to ask your doctor about ordering a blood test to see where you stand. You'll want the test that measures 25-hydroxyvitamin D, also called a 25(OH)D test. Don't bother with a test for 1,25-dihydroxyvitamin D. There's even a home test for 25(OH)D available from ZRT Laboratory. Order it online at *www.zrtlab.com.* Just prick your finger for a drop of blood, place it on special blotting paper, and return it to the lab for results.

B vitamins earn A+ for heart health

A bevy of B vitamins offer benefits like lowering cholesterol, preventing heart attacks, and avoiding stroke — but only if you get enough in supplements. Getting them only from food sources just won't do. Be sure to pick the right B vitamin for your particular need.

Cancel out high cholesterol with niacin. Also known as vitamin B3, you may hear niacin called by its active ingredient — nicotinic acid. You'll find it in many foods, including meat, fish, eggs, yeast, green vegetables, and cereals.

But as a supplement, large doses of niacin work to control high cholesterol. It's been shown to lower triglycerides by 20 to 30 percent and "bad" LDL cholesterol by as much as 20 percent. Even more important for certain people, niacin can raise "good" HDL cholesterol by nearly one-third. Niacin works by keeping your liver from producing too much very low-density lipoproteins (VLDL), which function like tiny suitcases to carry triglycerides through your bloodstream.

Successful tests used between 500 and 3,000 milligrams (mg) of niacin a day. Researchers say at doses of 1,000 to 2,000 mg, significant increases in HDL may occur. A dose of 1,000 mg of an extended-release niacin supplement helps improve blood vessel function. Niacin may also stave off other heart-related ills, like atherosclerosis — hardening of the arteries — and prevent a second heart attack.

Your doctor can prescribe niacin in two forms — Niacor (immediate release) or Niaspan (extended release). Although you can also buy niacin without a prescription, check with your doctor before you try it.

Combining niacin with a statin has an even more powerful effect than the supplement alone — lowering LDL cholesterol and triglycerides and raising HDL cholesterol. That's why some drug manufacturers are producing pills that contain both a statin and niacin. If you take a statin to lower your cholesterol, ask your doctor about this kind of combo pill, like lovastatin-niacin (Advicor) or simvastatin-niacin (Simcor).

Sidestep stroke with B-vitamin cocktail. Look to vitamin B6, vitamin B12, and folic acid to help prevent stroke. The Heart Outcomes Prevention Evaluation 2 study, nicknamed HOPE 2, found that people with heart disease may avoid stroke by taking a combination of these three B vitamins in supplements. The best stroke protection happened in people who took 2.5 mg folic acid, 50 mg vitamin B6, and 1 mg vitamin B12 every day.

This was especially true among people younger than age 69 and those from countries that don't enrich their food supply with folic acid. In 1998, the U.S. Food and Drug Administration ruled that manufacturers had to fortify grain-based foods with folic acid.

But not all studies find convincing benefits from taking B vitamins. In fact, the American Heart Association no longer recommends that everyone take B vitamins just to prevent heart disease.

Calm niacin's troubling side effects

Common side effects of taking niacin supplements include face flushing, itchiness, and rash. Try these tricks to avoid the side effects.

- Take an aspirin or ibuprofen one-half hour before you take your niacin supplement.

- Eat a snack with your supplement.

- Avoid hot baths or showers within an hour of taking the supplement.

- Take niacin at bedtime.

- Start with a low dose, then gradually increase to the prescribed dose.

- Try an extended-release version.

An oil more powerful than fish oil

Take a step farther down the food chain from fish oil, and you get to krill oil. This amazing oil helps your body in ways similar to fish oil — but it's even more powerful.

Krill oil is extracted from Antarctic krill, tiny crustaceans that are a food source for baleen whales, fish, and certain seabirds. Some people say krill oil supplements are more palatable than fish oil, with no fishy aftertaste. Like fish oil, krill oil contains eicosapentaenoic acid (EPA) and docosahexaenoic acid (DHA) — two important omega-3 fatty acids. But krill oil is a better source of these omega-3s than regular fish oil, and it also has vitamin A, vitamin E, and protein. It also provides astaxanthin, the pinkish-red antioxidant compound that gives the pink tint to shrimp and salmon.

Early research shows the omega-3 fatty acids in krill oil are more easily absorbed by your body than regular fish oil. The oil also does great things for your health.

High cholesterol. People with high cholesterol found that krill oil worked better than fish oil to lower cholesterol. In the study, participants taking 3 grams of krill oil daily lowered their "bad" LDL cholesterol by nearly 40 percent, while also lowering total cholesterol and triglycerides and raising "good" HDL cholesterol. Other research confirmed how krill oil can lower cholesterol.

Heart disease and arthritis. A study in people with heart disease and arthritis, either osteoarthritis or rheumatoid arthritis, found that those who took 300 milligrams of krill oil every day for just two weeks had lower levels of C-reactive protein, a marker of chronic inflammation. They also had improvements in their arthritis symptoms. Experts think the particular combination of omega-3 fatty acids and astaxanthin in krill oil blocked the inflammation.

Colon cancer. Lab tests using human colon cancer cells showed krill oil stopped their growth. Experts think four fatty molecules in krill oil block cancer — EPA, DHA, and alpha-linolenic acid (ALA), along with fatty molecules called sphingolipids.

You can find krill oil capsules, often called Neptune krill oil, at health food stores or online. Common brands include Jarrow, Nature's Way, and Source Naturals. A typical dose is 1 to 3 grams a day.

Krill oil may cause diarrhea or indigestion in some people. Beware of taking it if you're allergic to shellfish because you may also be allergic to krill oil. If you take blood thinners, krill oil may increase the effects of these drugs.

Go high-test for high triglycerides

Fish oil capsules are available over the counter and by prescription. Some people need the prescription-strength version. Super-potent fish oil capsules — brands like Omacor and Lovaza — cost about $160 a month. Not everyone needs them, but if your triglyceride level is very high, you'll benefit from this treatment. Four high-strength capsules provide 4,000 milligrams (mg) of omega-3 fatty acids. This high-strength omega-3 source is also commonly used in Europe alongside drugs to prevent a second heart attack.

Before you choose this pricey option, keep this in mind. Most people with heart disease need only three or four regular fish oil capsules daily, for around $10 a month. As with all over-the-counter supplements, buyer beware. Look for "USP Verified" on the label. That shows the product was tested for purity and strength by the U.S. Pharmacopeia.

5 popular herbs and how they help

Certain herbs can lower your cholesterol and help prevent stroke and heart failure. Yet, they carry a common risk — lack of regulation. Without knowing exactly how much you're getting in an herbal supplement, you risk taking too much or not enough to treat your condition. But if you're eager to try an herbal remedy, here are a few that have tested well. Talk to your doctor before you try one, especially if you're taking prescription drugs.

Ginkgo battles stroke. Ginkgo biloba comes from the ginkgo tree, which is considered sacred in China. Taking ginkgo daily may help prevent damage to your brain if you have a stroke. This herb also works to fight leg pain from blocked arteries, a condition called claudication.

Researchers continue to study ginkgo's effect on cerebral insufficiency, a condition caused by clogged blood vessels resulting in decreased blood flow to the brain. It shows up as problems concentrating, confusion, physical weakness, fatigue, headache, dizziness, depression, and anxiety. Ginkgo is a blood thinner, so don't take it if you have a bleeding or clotting problem, are taking warfarin (Coumadin), or are planning surgery.

Hawthorn douses heart failure. Made from dried flowers, fruit, and leaves of the hawthorn bush, this herbal extract is a popular treatment for congestive heart failure. Studies show it works, especially when you take hawthorn alongside drugs to improve heart function. Hawthorn also helps people who have congestive heart failure exercise longer and harder, because it boosts the amount of blood that reaches the heart.

Chia lowers cholesterol. Chia contains fiber and alpha-linolenic acid, a healthy fat. It may help lower triglycerides and raise "good"

HDL cholesterol. Mix chia seeds with water and you'll get a gel you can add to food or drinks.

Artichoke leaf extract lowers cholesterol. Antioxidant-rich artichokes are good for you, but an extract from the plant's leaves may be even better for you if you have high cholesterol. This extract is a traditional treatment in Europe to stimulate the kidneys and liver. Research shows artichoke leaf extract may also bring down high cholesterol.

Red yeast rice fights heart attack. This common ingredient in Chinese cooking is rice that's been fermented in a certain type of yeast. It's believed to lower cholesterol and reduce the risk of having a second heart attack.

Several years ago, the U.S. Food and Drug Administration (FDA) ordered some manufacturers to stop selling it because it contains monocolin A, the same active ingredient in the popular statin drug lovastatin. The FDA is also worried because dosages in over-the-counter red yeast rice supplements are not always reliable. Many experts suggest you stick with the well-regulated prescription statin.

Healthful living

4 tiny changes = 14 more years of fun

Is it possible to lower blood pressure, cholesterol, and blood sugar without expensive drugs? The experts say yes, and all it takes is four small changes.

These good-health behaviors are things you probably already know you should be doing. Researchers wanted to find out how helpful simple activities like eating right and exercising really are. They followed more than 20,000 people for a decade to see how they benefited from taking care of themselves. By the end of the study, the experts decided those men and women who practiced all four of the good-health behaviors were actually 14 years younger on the inside than people who didn't practice any of them.

Your heart, in particular, benefits from these changes, which don't require expensive drugs. People who practiced the good-health habits had fewer heart disease-related deaths than others. Other research shows taking care of yourself for just 12 weeks — paying attention to what you eat, getting active, and avoiding bad habits like smoking — can help you lower your blood pressure, choles-terol, and blood sugar. Here's all you need to do.

Eat your veggies. When you get at least five servings a day of fruits and vegetables, it shows. One sign scientists recognize is a high level of vitamin C in your blood. Getting the right nutrients helps your body fight off disease, including cancer. Fresh produce also gives you fiber, healthy phytochemicals — natural plant chemicals — and important vitamins and minerals. These can help keep your blood pressure, cholesterol, and blood sugar within a healthy range.

Get out and get active. Even people who hate the thought of working up a sweat can stay in good physical condition by adding fun forms of activity to their lives. Take the stairs instead of the elevator, give your flower garden a makeover, or go on a nature hike with your grandson.

People in the healthy-habits study scored best if they either were physically active at their jobs or spent at least 30 minutes a day doing something fun like swimming, dancing, or riding a bike. Exercise is good for your heart. Being overweight can bring on inflammation in your body, putting your heart in danger from high blood pressure, diabetes, and congestive heart failure.

Kick the habit. Smoking is a major factor in lung cancer, and it's also bad for your heart. People in the healthy-habits study who smoked were nearly twice as likely to die of heart-related problems as those who didn't smoke.

Keep alcohol within limits. Drinking too much alcohol is also harmful to your heart and may contribute to cancer. If you drink, limit it to no more than one drink a day for a woman or two drinks a day for a man. One drink equals a 12-ounce bottle of beer, a 4-ounce glass of wine, or a 1 1/2-ounce shot of 80-proof spirits. They all contain the same amount of alcohol.

Recover faster from a stroke

A little physical activity can help put your body on the road to recovery after a stroke. Researchers found that exercise, including walking on a treadmill and learning tai chi, may help improve walking and balance after a stroke. But don't wait until after the fact to get moving. People who stay physically fit tend to have less damage and recover better if they do suffer a stroke. So get up, get out, and protect your heart and your brain.

Fun way to turn back the clock

You'll love how easy it can be to stay young and healthy with a single anti-aging stunner. It's not a potion or pill, but simply keeping your body moving. A little physical activity a few times a week does it.

Experts did research on twins to see how their habits impact aging. Twin studies let researchers examine how different environments affect people with the same genetic makeup. The researchers found that twins who spend more of their leisure time doing physical activity have cells that age more slowly, based on looking at their chromosomes. The most active people got upward of three hours of exercise a week, while the least active clocked only 16 minutes a week.

These results were credited to more inflammation and oxidative stress in the body, along with more psychological stress, when people don't stay active. The study authors point out their results support recommendations for 30 minutes a day of moderate physical activity on at least five days of the week.

So how did these scientists figure the speed of aging? They measured the length of leukocyte telomeres, or chromosomes in white blood cells, of the twins. Actually, the telomeres are on the ends of chromosomes, kind of like the plastic tips on shoelaces that keep them from unraveling. Shorter telomeres are signs of diseases related to oxidative stress in your body, including heart disease, diabetes, and osteoporosis. More physical activity meant less risk for these conditions. And the researchers equated the amount of chromosome shortening to being 10 years younger in exercisers than nonexercisers.

Other studies have shown exercise encourages your body to build new blood vessels so your heart can handle the extra workload. Here's how you can help your heart with many types of activities. Just remember — always talk to your doctor before you start a new exercise program.

Get your blood pumping. When middle-age people take part in vigorous exercises, like running, they are healthier and live longer. But you don't have to knock yourself out to do your heart good. Researchers in Austria wanted to see whether hiking downhill is as good for you as hiking uphill. It is. People who hiked downhill several times a week for two months got the same health benefits, in terms of lower cholesterol and improved insulin resistance, as people who did more difficult uphill hiking. The researchers suggest easier downhill activity may be a good choice for people who can't do strenuous exercise, like those who are obese or who have congestive heart failure.

Light to moderate exercise, such as walking a few blocks or gardening, also lowers your risk of atrial fibrillation, a common heart arrhythmia in people over age 65.

Relax with tai chi. The ancient Chinese practice of tai chi, which involves gentle stretching, holding certain postures, and rhythmic movements, improves flexibility, balance, and strength. Studies show it also lowers blood pressure, improves cholesterol levels, and benefits people with congestive heart failure.

Pump some iron. If you have high blood pressure and you've always thought weight training was dangerous, think again. Now experts say that, although your numbers may rise while you lift weights, in the long run this kind of exercise can actually improve your blood pressure. That's because stronger muscles mean your heart doesn't have to work so hard. Go for a series of curls and presses two or three times a week.

You don't have to spend a lot of money to get fit.

- Spend less than $20 on a pedometer, and walk, walk, walk. People wearing a pedometer tend to walk an extra one to two miles a day.

- Get a jump-rope for less than $10, and exercise in the privacy of your own home.

- Don't buy weights when you can use your body. Do sit-ups, push-ups, and squats. Or grab those heavy cans of veggies from the pantry for strength training.

- Stop fighting traffic and bad weather if you enjoy cycling. Spend less than $100 on a trainer and turn your bike into a stationary cycle.

Heal yourself with music

Plug in to some Bach or Beatles, and your heart will happily sing along. Listening to music is a low-cost, drug-free way to stay healthy. It wakes up your body's natural healing ability to help you fight off disease.

A study of people with high blood pressure showed great results. When they listened to music for about a half-hour daily while practicing slow, deep-breathing exercises, their blood pressure went down. The researchers tried rhythmic classical, Celtic, or Indian music in the four-week study. People had an average drop in systolic blood pressure of about 4 mmHg. Other research found similar results.

Listening to music is a great stress reliever, and some experts think it works so well it can help keep you young. Long-term stress can break down your immune system, so doing something to avoid stress may boost your immunity. Researchers say listening to music you're especially fond of may really do the trick. It helps you relax, so blood vessels expand to let blood flow more smoothly. That's the same thing that happens when you laugh or take a statin drug.

Make your own music, and you'll really see some benefits. You don't have to take up playing an instrument — just hum a happy tune. It's the easiest health-booster ever.

How does it work? When you hum, your body's cells release nitric oxide, a gas that works in your brain to calm you down. That's why some experts suggest you try humming when you face a stressful event, like getting your blood drawn or having a flu shot. Believe it or not, researchers tested just how much more nitric oxide you produce when you hum compared to when you breathe out silently. They found you make about 15 times as much of this safe, natural body chemical.

Nitric oxide also helps your blood vessels relax, or dilate, so blood can flow more easily and your blood pressure goes down. Getting this nitric oxide boost by humming will also improve your immunity and calm your mind — plus it clears your sinuses. And you can do it anywhere.

Sound strategy for stroke victims

A stroke causes a blood clot or bleeding in the brain. That can stop you from walking, talking, and moving your body. Music may help you regain these abilities.

Singing may help you learn to speak again if this ability is damaged by stroke, a problem called aphasia. Damage to Broca's area of the brain — the speaking center in the left hemisphere — can take away your ability to talk. Singing therapy, or melodic intonation therapy, lets you use the undamaged part of your brain — in the right hemisphere where your musical ability lies — for tapping out rhythms, then singing, and eventually speaking.

And listening to pleasant music may help you regain vision after a stroke, probably because it improves your mood and lets you relax and focus better.

4 little-known ways to lower blood pressure

You can help lower your blood pressure with these four easy tips — whether or not your doctor has prescribed high blood pressure drugs. Keep in mind you should never stop taking a drug your doctor prescribed without his approval.

Make time for massage. Getting a massage may feel like the height of extravagance, but it's not all frivolous. Massage done by a trained massage therapist has definite health benefits. This simple touch therapy lowers your blood pressure while it boosts your immunity, eases pain, and reduces fatigue.

New research shows Swedish massage — a traditional style of massage using comfortable pressure to knead muscles — can lower your blood pressure. Other types of massage, like pressure-point massage, may actually do just the opposite. The key seems to be that you're relaxed, comfortable, and not in pain during the massage.

How does it work? Massage therapists say it works by bringing forth the relaxation response and increasing blood flow throughout your body. Those changes help decrease your blood pressure.

Consider a chiropractor. Adjustment of the C-1 vertebra or Atlas vertebra, the doughnut-shaped bone at the very top of your spine, may lower high blood pressure. Research shows people who had a chiropractor adjust this bone had lower blood pressure by 14 points systolic — the first number in the reading — and 8 points diastolic after eight weeks. That's as good as you get from taking two blood pressure medicines.

Chiropractors call the Atlas vertebra the body's "fuse box" because its location lets it control important body processes. That's why it's related to blood pressure, along with muscle and nerve function. Experts say getting help from a chiropractor may be a good option, especially if you've had head or neck trauma.

Watch the weather. Researchers in France found that seniors, especially those older than 80 years, tend to have seasonal variations in blood pressure. Both systolic and diastolic numbers were higher by an average of 5 points in winter than in summer. The change may be due to your body's efforts to keep warm by constricting blood vessels. Experts think this variation may explain the well-known higher risks of stroke and aneurysm during winter.

Track the changes. In one study, keeping track of their blood pressure helped people bring down their numbers over time. Researchers found this out when they gave wallet cards to veterans with high blood pressure, asking them to track changes and take certain steps to lower blood pressure.

Why you should say no to OTC cold medicines

Some cold medicines are bad for your heart. The pseudoephedrine in some nasal decongestants, like Sudafed, and cough syrups, such as Robitussin PE, works by constricting blood vessels in your nose. But the effect doesn't stop there. It can raise your blood pressure and heart rate. In rare cases, it can bring on an irregular heartbeat or even stroke. If you have health problems, talk to your doctor before you take an over-the-counter cold medicine.

Instead, open your nasal passages by standing in a hot shower. And coughing up phlegm is usually a better cure for congestion than suppressing the cough.

---

5 ways to avoid varicose veins

Those gnarled, swollen veins you can see through your skin are more than just unsightly. They're varicose veins, and they can be a sign of circulation problems. Varicose veins occur when weak valves in your leg veins let blood pool rather than return on the uphill trip to your heart. They may simply be unattractive, or they may cause pain, blood clots, or skin ulcers. Make these changes to keep your legs young and lovely at any age.

- Don't wear high heels. Almost all women make the mistake of wearing high heels sometimes. They can lead to varicose veins and back problems. That's because your calf muscles contract when you're in heels. Instead, stick with low-heeled shoes that help tone your calf muscles to encourage blood to move freely through your veins.

- Don't cross your legs, especially for long periods of time. This may raise your risk for varicose veins. When your legs remain in one position for a long time, veins must work harder to pump blood to your heart.

- Keep your legs active and your muscles strong to improve circulation in your legs. Try walking, climbing stairs, or dancing whenever you get the chance.

- Lose weight if you need to. This will improve circulation and ease stress on your veins.

- Avoid tight clothes, especially around your waist, groin, and legs.

Take 3 steps for everyday heart health

Taking care of your heart should be something you do every day. These three steps don't take much time, but they'll go a long way toward keeping your heart, and the rest of you, young and strong.

Walk yourself young. Exercise improves your cardiovascular fitness at any age. A number of studies show brisk walking benefits seniors by helping their hearts function like they're younger — even 12 years younger. This kind of activity boosted oxygen intake by about 25 percent. Seniors who went from sedentary to vigorous walking for about 45 minutes four times a week had improvements in their cardiovascular fitness similar to the benefits seen in younger people.

People who stay active by brisk walking, swimming, biking, or hiking for more than 60 minutes a week also suffer less disability as they age. A regular walking program reduces your chances of developing metabolic syndrome, a combination of risk factors for diabetes and heart disease that includes high blood pressure, obesity, and high cholesterol and blood sugar. Work on speeding up your walking pace and you'll increase your chances of living longer.

Walking is especially good if you suffer from peripheral arterial disease (PAD), blocked arteries in your legs that can cause pain. Giving your legs a workout may help develop collateral circulation, or the growth of alternative vessels to supply blood to muscles as they work.

Get your 40 winks. Balance all that exercise with the right amount of sleep. Too little sleep, less than six hours a night, or too much, more than eight hours, boosts your risk for metabolic syndrome. The ideal amount of sleep for adults is between seven and eight hours. Various studies have linked lack of sleep with higher body weight, inflammation, and diabetes. Too little sleep, even just a few hours, triggers inflammation in your body. That causes damage to healthy tissues and increases your risk of heart disease.

Laugh off stress. Job stress, traffic jams, money problems — all are bad for your heart. These events and your reactions to them put you in line for heart disease and a heart attack. A negative attitude causes your body to use up its heart-healthy antioxidant stores, increasing oxidative stress and damage to cells.

But research found watching at least one-half hour of funny videos or television every day counteracted the effects of stress, especially for people who had type 2 diabetes. Their HDL cholesterol level increased and blood levels of certain chemicals that incite inflammation decreased after the humor sessions. So give your heart something to laugh about.

Be kind to your heart with a HEPA filter

Spend a little money on an air filter, and your heart will breathe a sigh of relief. Exposure to air pollution raises your risk for heart disease, stroke, and deep vein thrombosis (DVT). But researchers found that seniors who used an air purifier in their homes with a high efficiency particle air (HEPA) filter had better heart function.

They tested the seniors' microvascular function, or how well the inner lining of tiny blood vessels worked. Poor microvascular function is a marker for heart disease. HEPA filters used for just two days removed 60 percent of particles from indoor air and were related to an 8 percent improvement in microvascular function.

Try these steps to reduce air pollution in your home.

- Clean often, using a vacuum cleaner with a HEPA filter.

- Change the filters on your air conditioner, and use those with a rating of MERV 8 (Minimum Efficiency Reporting Value).

- Get an air purifier with a HEPA filter for your bedroom.

- Replace carpet with wood or tile flooring.

5 ways to strike back at stroke

You can stay healthy, even as you get older. Take these steps to avoid illness, stave off stroke, and stay sharp as a tack.

Get your numbers checked. High blood pressure, or hypertension, is the leading risk factor for stroke. It's called the "silent disease" because it typically has no symptoms at first. That means you'll need to get your blood pressure checked to see if you're at risk. If yours is higher than 140/90 mmHg during at least two doctor visits, you may have high blood pressure.

When your blood pressure is too high, your blood puts too much pressure on the walls of your arteries as it passes through, causing damage over time. High blood pressure can lead to heart disease, kidney disease, vision loss, and dementia.

High cholesterol is another important stroke risk factor. That's because a buildup of cholesterol in your arteries can block the flow of blood to your brain, leading to a stroke.

Watch the clock. If you are a woman, your stroke risk rises sharply when you hit menopause. A drop in your estrogen level means you're no longer protected from high cholesterol and other heart-related ills. Both men and women who reach age 55 double their risk of stroke with each decade that passes. When you reach that milestone, pay close attention to your other risk factors.

Listen up. Sudden hearing loss could be an early sign of impending stroke. Research shows a stroke is more likely among people who've had sudden hearing loss in the past couple years than among people with no hearing loss. Gradual hearing loss as you age is different.

Take warning from migraines. If you're one of those unfortunate people who get migraine headaches, you're also at high risk of developing blood clots in your veins, a condition called venous thrombosis. Although researchers aren't sure how migraines and venous thrombosis are connected, changes in blood vessels or blood flow in the brain could be to blame. Research shows women who get migraines with aura, or visual disturbances, are up to 10 times more likely to have a stroke than other women.

Aim for clean living. Leading an unhealthy lifestyle — smoking, drinking alcohol, skipping exercise, and not eating enough fruits and vegetables — doubles your risk of stroke. That's a set of risks you can control.

Relax your fist for an accurate blood test

Not that long ago, the nurse told you to make a fist and clench it hard before she drew blood. That was to make your veins pop up for easier access. But health experts say that's not the best way to get accurate results.

Studies show tightening your muscles causes them to pump out potassium, which gets into the blood being drawn. That will make your blood level of potassium appear to be too high, and your doctor may order more tests to rule out kidney disease or heart problems. It may also cause you to have surgery delayed or be taken off medicines that can cause high potassium levels as a side effect.

Little-known heart attack signs

Heart attacks are not always as dramatic as what you see on television. In fact, only half of people having a heart attack feel the classic severe chest pain. Look for these signs.

- Pain and discomfort in the center of your chest, possibly radiating to one or both arms or your back, neck, or jaw. The discomfort may feel like a crushing weight on your chest or a tingling numbness in your arm.

- Shortness of breath.

- Nausea or breaking out in a cold sweat.

- Heartburn. If it's severe, pressing, squeezing pain that lasts more than 5 to 10 minutes, it's more likely to be a heart attack.

Women may just feel nauseous, have shortness of breath, and back or jaw pain instead of the classic symptoms.

If you think you may be having a heart attack, play it safe. Chew a 325-milligram aspirin and call 911.

Improve your stroke survival IQ

Don't ignore the warning signs of a stroke. If you act fast, you can avoid long-term damage or even save a life.

Strokes are the leading cause of disability and third-leading cause of death in the United States. Yet, most people aren't concerned about having one.

Strokes come in two forms — ischemic, when a blood clot blocks the blood supply to your brain, and hemorrhagic, or bleeding in your brain. Either way, brain cells don't get the oxygen they need, so they start dying off. This leads to brain damage. You may have heard of a mini-stroke, or transient ischemic attack (TIA). This happens when a blood clot temporarily blocks blood flow to your brain. It doesn't cause long-term damage, but it can be a warning sign of a future stroke.

Know the eight warning signs of stroke or TIA.

■ sudden weakness or numbness on one side of your face or one arm or leg

■ blurring, dimness, or loss of vision

■ memory loss or confusion

■ losing consciousness suddenly

■ slurred speech, inability to speak, or problems understanding other people

■ sudden, severe headache with no known cause

■ dizziness, drowsiness, lack of coordination, or falling

■ nausea and vomiting, especially when you also have other symptoms

If you or a loved one has these signs, take action fast. Here's what you should do immediately in case of a stroke.

Act quickly. Call 911. Make the person comfortable while you wait for an ambulance. Don't let her eat or drink. If an ambulance can't get there quickly, drive the person to the hospital.

Speed of treatment is important for the clot-busting drug t-PA, or tissue plasminogen activator, to help. It can lessen damage from an ischemic — but not hemorrhagic — stroke if given within three hours. A CT scan, done within 45 minutes of arriving in the ER, is the best way to tell if t-PA can help. Researchers are testing the cancer drug Bryostatin, which may prevent brain damage if given within the first 24 hours after a stroke.

Notify the stroke victim's doctor. This is important so the emergency team knows the person's medical history. At the hospital, share information on other conditions, like high blood pressure or diabetes, and medications.

'Shocking' way to save a life

Most victims of cardiac arrest die before emergency help arrives. In cardiac arrest, the heart stops beating because its electrical system malfunctions. Cardiac arrest often accompanies a heart attack, but sometimes seemingly healthy, young people experience this life-threatening emergency.

An automated external defibrillator (AED) can get the heart beating again. You may have seen AED boxes on the wall in airports, malls, and other public places. You can also buy one for your home, a good option if you're in a particular high-risk group. Ask your doctor if it's a good idea for you.

An AED is simple to use. The machine gives you directions when you open the box. It senses if the person needs an electrical shock to regain a normal heart rhythm. Get some training before an emergency so you'll be prepared.

Startling link between plastic containers and heart disease

You might want to give your body a breather from questionable plastics. Bisphenol A (BPA), a chemical used to make a hard plastic used in some water bottles and baby bottles, could spell trouble. Research suggests it can migrate into your food and may be linked to cancer. Now, scientists are finding connections between BPA and heart disease.

Research published in the *Journal of the American Medical Association* revealed that people with the most exposure to the chemical were at higher risk of having heart disease or diabetes. Exposure was determined by how much BPA appeared in urine. If this link proves true, it could be because BPA affects a hormone that protects against heart attacks and diabetes.

BPA may be linked to breast cancer, prostate cancer, and diabetes because of its estrogen-like effects. This connection to estrogen also seems to be at work in the heart. A recent study found that BPA combined with estrogen brought on heart arrhythmias, or an irregular heartbeat, in female mice. That's why experts worry about BPA's effects on the young, and authorities in Canada are considering banning the sale of BPA-containing baby bottles.

The U.S. Food and Drug Administration is reviewing evidence of BPA's dangers, but it hasn't yet banned it from food uses. Meanwhile, take these steps to lower your exposure.

- Don't use plastic containers to heat up food in the micro-wave — even those that claim to be microwave-safe. Chemicals may leach from the plastic into your food.

- Use glass, porcelain, or stainless-steel containers to hold food. Avoid hard plastics.

- Don't wash plastic containers in the dishwasher, where detergents may break down the plastic and release BPA.

■ Switch from canned to frozen or fresh vegetables to avoid BPA that may lurk in can linings.

■ Look for the claim "BPA free" on labels of water bottles and baby bottles. Or check the bottom of plastic bottles for the number "1" within a triangle. Avoid those with the number "7."

An aspirin a day keeps the doctor away

Sometimes the simplest and cheapest way is also the best. That may be true when it comes to drugs that protect your heart. Aspirin is a cheap, safe drug with many heart benefits. But it's not right for everyone.

The benefits. Daily low-dose aspirin therapy refers to taking between 75 to 100 milligrams (mg) of aspirin once a day. Benefits include preventing heart disease and stroke. In fact, many heart experts encourage people at high risk of these conditions to take low-dose aspirin daily, unless they have health problems that make it unsafe.

Aspirin can lower your blood pressure if you have prehypertension, or blood pressure that's just below the 140/90 cutoff mark for high blood pressure. But research shows you must take your low-dose aspirin at night, not in the morning, to get this blood pressure-lowering effect. The reason is unclear, but researchers think aspirin may be better absorbed from your digestive tract at night.

If you think you're having a heart attack, take a 325-mg aspirin and call 911. Chewable aspirin may be your best bet, since it's more easily absorbed. Aspirin is the best immediate treatment for acute coronary syndrome, a range of symptoms related to an insufficient amount of blood flowing to your heart, including angina and heart attack.

The risks. Aspirin's antiplatelet effect prevents blood clots, but it can cause bleeding in your digestive system. If you're healthy, many health professionals say you should wait to take daily aspirin until the benefits outweigh the risks. For men, that's usually after age 40. While for women, it's age 65. New research shows that only people who have heart disease should take daily aspirin. Be sure to talk with your doctor before you begin daily aspirin therapy.

Don't mix aspirin with other pain relievers like ibuprofen (Advil, Motrin), which can block aspirin from doing its job. Some experts say you can take aspirin, wait at least four hours, then take your other pain reliever to avoid this interaction.

Wonder drug cuts cholesterol

Statins work. They can lower your high cholesterol and cut your risks of further heart damage after a heart attack. But they're not a magic pill for everyone.

How they help. You've probably heard of drugs like Zocor, Crestor, and Lipitor. They can lower your "bad" LDL cholesterol to cut your risk of heart attack and stroke. If you take a statin after you've had a heart attack, you reduce your chances of dying by 25 to 30 percent.

Statins work by blocking a liver enzyme called HMG-CoA reductase, which your body needs to make cholesterol. When your liver isn't making its own cholesterol, your body takes it from your blood and uses it for building hormones and other important functions. Statins also lower triglycerides and raise your levels of "good" HDL cholesterol.

There are also hints statins may protect your heart if you have diabetes, reduce your likelihood of having a stroke, lower high blood pressure, and protect against kidney disease. Beyond that, they may stave off liver cancer and reduce the need for gallbladder removal.

A recent study, called the Jupiter study, suggests statin benefits for people who don't have high cholesterol. Researchers took a group of healthy people with normal cholesterol levels in their 50s and

60s and tested their levels of C-reactive protein (CRP). A high CRP level shows you're at higher risk for heart attack. Of the people with a high CRP, half started taking statins and half took a placebo, or sugar pill. Those on statins lowered their risk of heart attack by 54 percent, stroke by 48 percent, and the need for bypass surgery or angioplasty by 46 percent.

Consider the side effects. Many experts warn these results don't mean statins should be prescribed to all people. First, they're expensive. You could spend more than $1,200 a year for a name-brand drug like rosuvastatin (Crestor).

More importantly, statins can cause serious side effects, especially the more powerful drugs. The most dangerous risk is rhabdomyolysis, or a breakdown of muscle fibers. This releases a protein called myoglobin into your bloodstream, where it can travel to your kidneys and cause kidney damage. Muscle breakdown is rare, but it can be deadly if it's not caught early.

There are other possible side effects, and not all doctors are aware of them.

■ Problems with memory and thinking. Your brain needs cholesterol to build neurotransmitters that allow brain cells to communicate. Without enough cholesterol, brain function may suffer.

■ Peripheral neuropathy, or pain and numbness in your fingers and toes.

■ Higher blood sugar levels and tendon problems.

Scientists think these side effects are caused by changes in your mitochondria, the energy-producing "power plant" of cells. These changes seem to lead to an increase in damaging free radicals in your body. It's possible to experience one of these side effects suddenly, even if you've been on a statin safely for years. The risks increase with age.

Many experts say you should change your behavior through healthy eating and regular exercise if you want to cut your heart disease risk and lower your cholesterol. Don't rush to take statins if you're not at risk.

Beware of dangerous drug combo

Don't take Prilosec (omeprazole) or most other proton-pump inhibitors for heartburn if you're taking Plavix (clopidogrel) to prevent a second heart attack. New research shows this combination raises your risk of another heart attack.

Most proton-pump inhibitors block the liver's ability to change Plavix to its active form, which is essential to prevent blood clots from forming. These two drugs are among the most commonly prescribed drugs in the world, so the chance of being on both is pretty high.

If you're taking Plavix and have trouble with too much stomach acid, ask your doctor about taking other drugs, like Zantac (ranitidine) or Protonix (pantoprazole), which don't raise your heart attack risk.

When you can safely bypass a bypass

Angioplasty or coronary bypass surgery — which is right for you? A less-invasive procedure costs less and may mean quicker recovery time. That's a great reason to ask your doctor about angioplasty and stents if she suggests you have coronary bypass surgery. You'll have less trauma, pain, expense, and time in the hospital — if angioplasty is right for you.

Angioplasty, also known as percutaneous coronary intervention, is a procedure to open up clogged arteries that supply blood to your heart. These arteries can become blocked with fatty deposits and fibrous tissue known as plaque. With angioplasty, a surgeon uses a catheter to inflate a balloon inside the clogged artery, sometimes also placing a stent, or tiny tube, to keep the artery open. Unlike with bypass surgery, angioplasty doesn't require that your chest and heart be opened up.

When angioplasty is done to clear blocked arteries soon after a heart attack, the procedure can save a life. It also may put an end to stable angina, or chest pain that occurs with exercise or stress but goes away on its own.

Angioplasty is not as helpful as a preventive measure. Some experts say that's partly because when plaque builds up the buildup occurs in more than one or two places. That means plaque buildup needs to be resolved in all affected areas, using the gentler remedies of a healthy diet, regular exercise, and drugs.

In fact, for people with stable angina, using drugs alone may work as well as angioplasty or stents, although it may take longer to open up clogged arteries. One study found adding angioplasty to drug therapy didn't decrease heart attack risk or increase life span in these people. In other words, either treatment gave good results. Drug therapy in this case consisted of aspirin, statins, beta-blockers, blood vessel dilators, and various clot-busting drugs.

Yet, sometimes bypass is the way to go. One study found that people with severe heart disease — those with at least three clogged coronary arteries or a single clog in the left main artery — had more success with bypass surgery than with stents. That means they had less chance of an artery clogging up again and lower risk of another heart attack, stroke, or need for a repeat procedure. Only about 5 percent of people who receive stents in the United States fall into this group.

Rethink surgery to sidestep superbugs

Here's another reason to rethink surgery — having an invasive procedure and more time in the hospital means a higher risk of picking up a deadly superbug infection.

Bacteria are everywhere, but certain drug-resistant strains or superbugs, like *Clostridium difficile (C. difficile)* and methicillin-resistant *Staphylococcus aureus* (MRSA), are more common in hospital settings. The U.S. Centers for Disease Control (CDC) says as many as 1.7 million people pick up infections in the hospital every year.

One common danger is a central line bloodstream infection, caused by bacteria invading a tube that delivers medication directly into a vein. Fortunately, these infections are preventable. Hospital workers should use good hygiene, like washing their hands, using sterile drapes, and carefully cleaning a patient's skin with chlorhexidine soap before inserting a tube.

Unfortunately, regular routine cleaning won't kill some superbugs. One study found 78 percent of hospital surfaces were still contaminated after routine cleaning. Using a checklist can work to cut infections, but many hospitals don't always follow the safest practices.

Take these steps to keep yourself safe in the hospital.

■ Choose wisely. Do some research to pick the local hospital with the best infection history. Get information on hospitals in your area at *www.StopHospitalInfections.org* or *www.SafePatientProject.org*. Hospitals in 25 states are required to make their infection rates public.

■ Before a nurse or doctor touches you, insist that they wash their hands thoroughly using soap and water. They should also clean their stethoscopes between patients.

- Wash your hands before you eat. Don't touch your mouth or eyes.

- Ask your family to bring in wipes containing bleach to clean surfaces in your hospital room and items around the bed.

- Beware of certain medications, including antibiotics and heartburn drugs. Antibiotics can kill off your helpful bacteria, increasing your chances of colonization by *C. difficile*. Heartburn drugs block stomach acid, which helps keep bacteria under control. This also increases your risk of infection.

- After you get home from the hospital, assume anything you brought with you is contaminated. Wash your hospital laundry separately using bleach.

Pneumonia vaccine blocks heart attacks

Take her advice if your doctor suggests you get a vaccination to prevent pneumonia. You may also be protecting yourself from a heart attack.

A recent study shows that people who received the pneumonia vaccination within the past two years had a 50 percent lower risk of having a heart attack. Experts aren't sure why, but they think the vaccine's effect on your immune system also blocks inflammation of the coronary arteries that supply blood to your heart. Less inflammation means less risk of heart attack.

Safeguard your bones & joints

New twist on bone loss

Remember mixing vinegar and baking soda when you were a child? You got a wonderful bubbling fizz the moment the acid in the vinegar met the alkaline compounds in baking soda. But chemistry doesn't just happen in a glass. Acid and alkaline compounds from foods may also affect your bones.

How it works. When you eat, your body converts food into compounds it can use for fuel. Eating lots of meat and cereal grains produces acids in your body. This happens because some minerals, like the sulfur hidden in meat proteins, break down into acids when you digest them. So does the phosphorous lurking in cereal grains.

As you age, your body has a tougher time getting rid of all those acids, so they build up. The acids muzzle your bone-making cells, while revving up cells that remove bone. To neutralize those acids, your body may steal calcium, phosphates, and alkaline compounds from your bones — making them weaker. When you eat more fruits and vegetables, your body ends up with more alkaline compounds, and your skeleton can keep its calcium.

Examine the evidence. In a recent study from Tufts University, older adults who took an alkaline supplement lost less calcium than people who didn't take the supplement. To be sure their results were accurate, the researchers also tested for a compound called NTX. The more NTX your body makes, the more bone you are probably losing. The researchers discovered that people who took alkaline supplements had lower NTX levels than people who didn't take the supplements.

If you'd like to get results like these, aim for plenty of servings of fruits and veggies every day. According to the researchers, eating lots of fruits and veggies may give you the same results as taking an alkaline supplement.

5 powerful ingredients for a bone-boosting salad

The best osteoporosis defense is a good offense. Don't just add more fruits and veggies to your diet. Choose the ones armed with extra skeleton-saving compounds to help keep your bones stronger for longer. Here are five delicious, bone-building ways to add zip to a salad.

Start with a great green, like spinach. Popeye's favorite food — spinach — is a great source of vitamin K. Some studies suggest your risk of fractures may go up if you don't get enough of this often-forgotten vitamin. To add even more vitamin K to your diet, cook up all-natural, leafy greens like kale, collard greens, and turnip greens. A word of caution — if you take a blood-thinning drug, like warfarin, talk to your doctor before adding more vitamin K to your diet. Vitamin K can interfere with these drugs.

Enjoy sun-dried tomatoes. This trendy version of the humble tomato contains loads of lycopene. An exciting, new study found that women who ate more lycopene had less bone loss from their spines than women who didn't. Lycopene seems to interfere with the birth of cells that break down bone. If you'd like more lycopene in your diet, enjoy more pasta sauces, tomato-based soups, and foods that contain cooked tomato, tomato puree, or tomato paste.

Add sweet red peppers. These tasty morsels offer a variety of carotenoids — lycopene, lutein, and zeaxanthin. Research suggests that men who eat more carotenoids, including lycopene, lutein, and zeaxanthin, may be better protected from bone loss in their hips. Gobble up more sweet red peppers, but don't stop there. Enjoy spinach, kale, turnip greens, peas, winter squash, pumpkin, corn, and collard greens — also great sources of lutein and zeaxanthin.

Rediscover dried plums. Add a dash of unexpected sweetness with diced dried plums. Earlier studies suggest the powerful polyphenols in these fruits may help fight osteoporosis. Now a recent lab study suggests that dried plum polyphenols may promote the formation of bone-making compounds and help your bone-making cells get the job done.

Top it off with olive oil. Make a great-tasting salad even better with an oil-and-vinegar dressing. Just make sure the oil is olive oil. A study of Greek men and women found that monounsaturated fats, like olive oil, may help your bones stay strong. What's more, an animal study found that tyrosol and other olive oil compounds might protect against bone loss. You need a little bit of oil to make sure your body absorbs the carotenoids. So be sure to drizzle oil-and-vinegar — with bone-healthy olive oil — on all your salads.

Invigorating brew beats brittle bones

Milk isn't the only bone-building beverage. Tea can help you battle osteoporosis, boost bones, and fend off fractures.

Tea helps because it has anti-aging abilities that directly affect your bones. Here's why. When you're younger, your body makes new bone faster than it can remove old, worn-out bone. But as you age, you begin losing bone faster than you can make it. Your bones become like a brick wall where the mortar is wearing away. Just as missing mortar makes the wall weaker, missing bone makes your skeleton more fragile. Your doctor may call this low bone mass or low bone mineral density (BMD). If your bones get weak enough, you can get disabling bone fractures or breaks. Fortunately, studies show how tea can help prevent this.

An Australian study of women over age 70 found that tea drinkers lost less bone mass over a four-year period than tea avoiders. Scientists think the flavonoids in tea may help rev up your bone-making cells so you make bone faster than you lose it. Drink four or more cups of your favorite black tea daily and studies suggest you'll increase your BMD. If you prefer an occasional cup of green tea, get your tea kettle ready. Green tea has also been linked to higher BMD and may even help prevent hip fractures.

Uncover the real truth about calcium

These two common mistakes could keep calcium from protecting you against fractures. Here's how to avoid them for stronger bones.

Getting too much. Experts say once you get enough calcium, adding more may not lower your fracture risk any further. Several studies have even suggested that people who take calcium supplements are no better protected from a hip fracture than people who don't take calcium supplements. Now, some experts think these studies may be wrong. In one study, many participants in both the "high calcium" and "low calcium" groups were already getting approximately 1,000 milligrams (mg) of calcium a day — close to the recommended amount. That may be why the extra calcium taken by the "high calcium" group didn't make much difference in fracture risk.

Many experts also warn that too much calcium could cause a short- age of the phosphorus you need to build bone. Health professionals suggest you aim for at least 1,200 mg a day if you are over age 50 and 1,500 mg if you have osteoporosis — but no more than 2,000 mg a day. Fortunately, it's tough to get too much calcium from foods, so try to get all you need from daily meals and snacks. For example, a cup of Total Raisin Bran can give you 1,000 mg of cal- cium without milk, or up to 1,290 mg with a cup of low-fat milk. Or enjoy an 8-ounce cup of yogurt and get 452 mg. Other good sources of calcium include ricotta cheese, sardines, chocolate milk, and buttermilk.

Ignoring salt intake. Make salt mistake and even calcium-rich foods and supplements may leave you calcium-poor. A British study found that women whose daily diets included two or more teaspoons of salt lost more calcium from their bodies than the 1,280 mg per day they took in. Not surprisingly, women who took in less salt did not develop this problem. Consider cutting back on salt by one-third and use spices to add flavor instead. But for even better results, get more potassium, too.

A California study found that women on a high-salt diet who got extra potassium lost far less calcium than women who got less potassium. The women in the high potassium group also showed signs of less bone loss. The University of California scientists say you can get as much potassium as the women in the study if you eat seven to eight servings of potassium-rich fruits and veggies every day. Consider rich sources like these — white beans, beet greens, dates, raisins, lima beans, spinach, papaya, and tomato sauce.

Build up your bones with mineral water

Milk may not always be your best source of calcium. The label may say 300 milligrams (mg) of calcium per serving, but how much you really get depends on something called bioavailability — or how easily your body can absorb and use a particular kind of calcium from a particular drink.

Research shows that your body can use more of the calcium from some drinks than from others. In other words, if two drinks promise 300 mg of calcium per serving, you'll get more calcium from the drink with high bioavailability than you will from the drink with low bioavailability.

Bioavailability	Drink
low	orange juice rice milk soy milk
medium	milk
high	high-calcium mineral water

Fight fractures with chili

A hearty bowl of chili can be perfect after traipsing through winter rain or snow. Not only does it chase away bone-chilling cold, it may help keep your bones strong — if you use the right ingredients. Here's what you'll need for bone-building chili. You'll find the recipe for "Anaheim Black Bean Chili" on the following page.

Black beans. These beans are rich in magnesium, a mineral your body needs to absorb calcium. In fact, if you get enough magnesium, you'll absorb extra calcium from the foods you eat — even if you don't add more calcium to your diet. Even better, studies hint that people who get more magnesium tend to have stronger bones.

Unfortunately, many older adults don't get enough magnesium. You may be one of them, especially if you have an irregular heartbeat or muscle cramps. If that's the case, consider adding magnesium-rich foods to your daily menu.

Good choices include halibut, Brazil nuts, pinto beans, white beans, okra, brown rice, and spinach. But be careful. If you regularly take large amounts of over-the-counter laxatives, antacids, or pain relievers, talk to your doctor before adding more magnesium to your diet. You may already get plenty of this mineral from these medications.

Lean ground beef. A meaty chili can give you extra vitamin B12, a vitamin that's difficult for most older adults to get enough of. Research shows that people with lower B12 levels have lower bone mass density, which means weaker bones.

Getting enough B12 helps your bone-making cells do their jobs. It also helps prevent an amino acid called homocysteine from interfering with the collagen that makes your bones strong. If ground beef doesn't appeal to you, you can get even more B12 from fortified cereals, shellfish, sardines, salmon, and other fish.

Anaheim Black Bean Chili

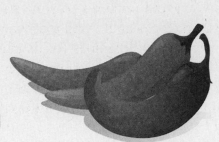

3 lbs. lean ground beef

4 cloves garlic, finely chopped

1 15-oz. can tomato sauce

2 teaspoons red chili powder

1 teaspoon ground cumin seed

1 teaspoon ground coriander

4 minced Anaheim or other chili peppers

1 15-oz. can black beans

3 cups of water

1 small can of tomato paste (optional)

1. Combine the ground beef and garlic. Simmer until the beef is brown. Remove the excess fat.

2. Add the tomato sauce and red chili powder.

3. Add the cumin seed, ground coriander, and Anaheim or other chili peppers, black beans, and water.

4. For thicker chili, add a small can of tomato paste or less water. For chili that's not as hot, use fewer peppers.

5. Bring all ingredients to a boil and turn down the heat to low. Simmer uncovered, stirring frequently, for about 30 minutes.

Serves 6 or more.

Turn back the clock on aging bones

A secret ingredient in peanuts and red grapes could be your ticket to stronger, more youthful bones. This incredible compound may help you avoid fractures so you can lead the life you want. Grape skins, grapes, peanuts, and red wine all contain resveratrol, a phytonutrient already famous for its ability to protect your heart. When researchers fed huge helpings of resveratrol to middle-age mice, they discovered that resveratrol helped prevent bone loss, too. Fortunately, resveratrol doesn't just work in mice.

Get the facts. A recent study suggests that people who drink a half or whole glass of red wine or another alcoholic beverage every day are 20 percent less likely to fracture a hip than those who don't drink at all. What's more, research from Tufts University found that older women who drank wine daily had stronger bones in their hips and spines than nondrinkers. The researchers suspect the anti-aging powers of wine's resveratrol may be the reason why.

Before menopause, women have enough estrogen in their bodies to help them make bone faster than they lose it. But after menopause, estrogen levels drop. Lower estrogen levels cause bone-making cells to work more slowly than the cells that remove old bone, so you lose bone faster than you can make it. Even when your estrogen levels drop, resveratrol can help because it has estrogen-like powers. Research suggests these estrogen-like powers may help prevent bone loss in women after menopause — which is almost like an anti-aging treatment for your skeleton.

Heed the warnings. Resveratrol's great study results don't mean you should take up drinking or increase your number of drinks a day. After all, alcohol consumption automatically raises your risk of fracture-causing falls, breast cancer, and cirrhosis of the liver. So what should you do? If you don't drink, don't start. Instead, add more grape juice and grapes to your diet since these are good sources of resveratrol. Also, enjoy these other good sources — peanuts and peanut butter.

People at high risk for heart disease may benefit from red wine, but those with a family history of breast cancer or other health problem may be better off not drinking alcoholic beverages. Before you pour yourself a glass of wine, weigh your health risks and discuss them with your doctor, especially if you take prescription drugs.

Warning for chocolate lovers

Chocolate really does go straight to your hips, but not in the way most people think. Australian researchers discovered that women who ate chocolate every day had weaker bones in their hips, shins, and heels. They also had poorer overall bone density. The scientists suspect sugar and a compound called oxalate may be the culprits.

Oxalate keeps your body from absorbing the calcium needed for strong bones, while sugar encourages your body to get rid of more calcium than usual. More research needs to be done, but if you're worried about osteoporosis, cut back on chocolate to just once a week.

Insider's scoop on soy and bones

News stories recently proclaimed that soy prevents bone loss in older women, but now the stories have changed. It's like watching a pendulum swing back and forth. Here's how you can make sense out of all the confusion.

Discover the secret behind isoflavones. The real skeleton-savers in soy are its isoflavone compounds, like genistein and daidzein. Studies suggest these compounds rev up your bone-making cells, while hampering the cells that destroy old bone. When you make bone faster and lose it more slowly, you keep more of your bone. Then again, many other studies hint that soy has no effect on bone loss.

Understand equol's role. Some experts think the secret is equol, a compound your body can make from daidzein. A preliminary laboratory study suggests that equol may limit the number of bone-destroying cells your body can make — and that can help you keep more of your bones for longer. Keep in mind that only 30 to 50 percent of people can make equol after eating soy, and finding out whether you're an equol maker is tough to do. However, one study suggests that women who eat more fiber, carbohydrates, and plant proteins are more likely to produce equol.

Research suggests that equol makers seem to benefit more from soy than people whose bodies can't make equol. And if the early studies are proven right, up to 50 percent of people may reduce bone loss by eating daidzein-containing soy foods, like tempeh, soy milk, and roasted or boiled soybeans. Of course, that only accounts for the effects of daidzein. Genistein may also work to save your bones. But no matter which isoflavone is responsible, the most important thing to remember is this — many randomized controlled trials, the most reliable kind of study, suggest that soy compounds slow bone loss. Soy may just make your bones act younger than their age.

Consider the side effects. Before you try soy, talk to your doctor because some forms of soy may raise your risk of dementia. For detailed information on how soy foods affect your brain, see "Smarter ways to enjoy soy" on page 15 in *Age-proof your brain*. If you decide to try soy, don't let that be your only path to better bones. Remember to get plenty of calcium and vitamin D, and make weight-bearing exercise a part of your routine.

Discover a unique bone builder

Silicon, a mineral found in beer, may be linked to higher bone mass in both men and women. Silicon may stimulate your body to make more collagen, a key substance that helps make your bones both flexible and strong. Since drinking alcohol can be hazardous to your health, consider getting your silicon from sources like unrefined whole grains, cereal, and root vegetables.

Survival guide for coffee drinkers

Coffee can be good or bad depending on whether you're worried about gout or osteoporosis. Here are some things to consider.

The Good. Men who drink coffee may lower their gout risk as much as 60 percent, a recent study suggests. Another study found that drinking at least four cups of coffee a day may significantly lower your risk of gout. Researchers think an antioxidant — chlorogenic acid — and other compounds in coffee may cut your uric acid levels. Less uric acid may mean you're in less danger of developing gout. This doesn't mean you should start drinking coffee if you've never been a java fan. But if you're a coffee lover who has gout or a high risk of getting it, go ahead and enjoy your cuppa joe.

The Bad. Some experts think consuming lots of caffeine, especially from coffee, may cause your body to lose more bone-building calcium. If they're right, too much coffee could raise your risk of bone loss and fractures. Although some studies hint that only thin, older women are truly at risk, more research is needed. Meanwhile, play it safe and ask your doctor how much caffeine you can safely drink.

The Ugly. If you take the bone-building drug alendronate (Fosamax) for osteoporosis, don't take it with coffee. Coffee can cripple your body's ability to absorb this medication — so you may get less medicine than you paid for, but more risk of bone loss and fractures. To prevent this, don't drink coffee within two hours of taking alendronate.

3 great reasons to get more vitamin C

Bypass fragile bones and painful joints by adding foods rich in vitamin C to your daily meal plan. This powerful antioxidant can help your bones and joints three ways.

Repels arthritis. If your doctor finds signs of degeneration in your knees, you're probably developing osteoarthritis. Amazingly, Australian researchers found that people who got the most vitamin C from their diets were less likely to have these signs. The same was true of people who ate lots of fruit. Why not be nice to your knees and try both? Good examples of fruits rich in vitamin C include papaya, oranges, kiwifruit, pineapple, and strawberries.

Prevents the raging pain of gout. A Boston University study found that men who took up to 1,500 milligrams (mg) of vitamin C supplements had as much as a 45 percent lower risk of developing gout compared with men who did not take supplements. The researchers think vitamin C fights both the inflammation and the high uric acid levels that contribute to gout.

Strengthens your bones. You might think vitamin D and calcium are the only nutrients that protect you against brittle bones. Yet, research shows that people who don't get enough vitamin C lose bone faster. Vitamin C helps protect your bones in two ways. It helps produce collagen, a compound that weaves into your bones to make them stronger, and it fights inflammation. That's good news because inflammation can trigger the removal of old bone and speed up bone loss.

Some experts say you can get enough vitamin C just by eating five servings of fruits and vegetables every day. But a recent study found that those who take vitamin C supplements are only half as likely to experience hip fractures as those who don't. The study also discovered that people who get the most vitamin C — from both foods and supplements — are only half as likely to fracture a hip as those who get the lowest amounts of vitamin C. The study participants who got the most vitamin C took in 305 mg, with 260 mg coming from supplements.

Get as much vitamin C from foods as you can to defend your bones and help prevent gout. Then talk to your doctor about whether you should take supplements.

Sweet relief for arthritis pain

Arthritis pain is the pits, so why not fight back with a bowl of cherries? Some experts think they may be as good as aspirin. Studies suggest that cherries have anti-inflammatory powers, just as aspirin does. Scientists can tell because the levels of certain compounds in your blood spike when inflammation is attacking your body. These include C-reactive protein (CRP), nitric oxide, and a compound nicknamed RANTES. Higher nitric oxide levels, in particular, have been associated with tissue damage in both osteoarthritis (OA) and rheumatoid arthritis, while higher RANTES levels have been linked to OA.

But a funny thing happened when researchers asked 20 people to eat 45 cherries a day for a month. Their CRP levels plummeted by

25 percent, their nitric oxide levels dropped by 18 percent, and their RANTES levels fell by 21 percent. Researchers think this means powerful compounds, called polyphenols, in cherries fight arthritis inflammation. Anthocyanins, a type of polyphenol, help give cherries their color.

Besides having anti-inflammatory powers, they are particularly good at squelching nitric oxide. They even attack the COX-1 and COX-2 compounds that help cause inflammation. In fact, some studies hint that anthocyanins may be as good at quenching these inflammatory compounds as over-the-counter painkillers, like ibuprofen, naproxen, and aspirin.

Yet, cherries don't just fight arthritis. Eating cherries also changes the faulty body chemistry behind gout, a type of arthritis. Doctors say gout is caused by too much uric acid in your bloodstream. That uric acid forms little needle-like crystals that sneak into your joints and cause inflammation and pain. But a study from the University of California at Davis found that women experienced a drop in uric acid after eating cherries. Their nitric oxide and CRP levels also fell. Lower levels of these compounds may mean less pain in your future.

If you'd like to add more cherries to your diet, sweet or tart cherries can both help, but tart cherries have more anthocyanins. Try dried cherries or cherry juice concentrate if you need cherries in a more concentrated form that's available year round.

Fight rheumatoid arthritis with fewer painkillers

Arthritis can make you feel as stiff as the rusted Tin Man from *The Wizard of Oz*. But why use an oil can when you can loosen your joints with a different kind of oil — the one found in fish. Studies show that the omega-3 fatty acids in fish oil are powerful anti-aging agents that can improve your joint mobility, while protecting you from arthritis.

What fish oil can do for you. British researchers asked 97 people with rheumatoid arthritis (RA) to take combination capsules of fish oil and cod liver oil every day for nine months. The capsules contained just over 2 grams of omega-3 fatty acids. At 12 weeks, they asked the study participants to gradually cut back on their nonsteroidal anti-inflammatory drugs (NSAIDs). Amazingly, nearly 40 percent were able to cut their NSAID use by more than a third without having their arthritis worsen. Researchers concluded that omega-3 fatty acids can fight the inflammation that causes RA symptoms.

Now the bad news. Omega-3s have an evil twin — the omega-6 fatty acids found in vegetable oil, red meat, and foods containing trans fats, like fried foods, margarine, and shortening. Unfortunately, most people eat far more omega-6 fatty acids than omega-3 fatty acids. Omega-6s promote inflammation in your body, so you need even more omega-3s to counteract them.

In fact, studies have found that RA inflammation can be suppressed if you get twice as many omega-3s as omega-6s. At least 13 studies have shown that omega-3 supplements can reduce pain and stiffness, as well as the number of painful joints associated with RA. What's more, you may get a bonus benefit from fish oil — improved brain function. A Norwegian study found that older adults who ate at least a third of an ounce of fish every day were more likely to score higher on learning, memory, perception, and judgment tests than people who ate less fish. Unprocessed lean fish and omega-3-loaded fatty fish were the most effective.

Safe way to eat more fish. Many health experts recommend eating at least two servings of fish every week, but don't go hog wild. Eating more than a few servings weekly could expose you to unsafe amounts of mercury, pesticides, and other toxins. Swordfish, shark, tilefish, and king mackerel are particularly dangerous, so avoid them. Stick with healthier choices, like salmon, shrimp, herring, and canned light tuna. To make fish more effective, many experts suggest cutting back or avoiding foods containing omega-6 fatty acids. If eating more omega-3 foods and less omega-6 foods doesn't help, try eliminating tomatoes, eggplant, peppers, and white potatoes and see if your symptoms improve. These foods aggravate inflammation in some people.

Help from supplements. You can't get all the fish oil needed to fight RA just by eating fish. Studies suggest you need about 2 grams of fish oil to get RA relief, but a serving of fish can't give you that much. Fortunately, independent testing shows that fish oil capsules are free of mercury, pesticides, and other toxins found in fish. Plus, you can get more omega-3s from the capsules than you're likely to get from fish. To get the most benefit, remember these tips.

- Start with smaller doses and take the supplements with meals to avoid unpleasant side effects, like gas, burping, or a fishy aftertaste.

- Check the dose per capsule to make sure you're getting the right amount of fish oil each day.

- Before you try these supplements, talk with your doctor. Fish oil supplements can thin your blood, so you shouldn't take them if you already take a blood thinner, such as warfarin.

Conquer RA with an amazing vitamin

Get enough vitamin D and you might avoid rheumatoid arthritis. A study of nearly 30,000 women suggests that women who get more of the "sunshine vitamin" have a lower risk of developing RA. Vitamin D may help your body resist RA by fighting inflammation and regulating your immune system.

4 tasty ways to tame inflammation

A tip from Smokey the Bear might help ease your arthritis symptoms. Smokey always said a spark is enough to start a forest fire. Likewise, sparks of inflammation in your joints trigger rheumatoid arthritis (RA) symptoms. Research suggests you may help dowse your symptoms if you eat inflammation-fighters like these.

- Fruits and veggies. Research shows that antioxidants battle inflammation. Good choices include apples, berries, broccoli, spinach, brussels sprouts, and kale.

- Olive oil. This oil contains omega-3 fatty acids and oleocanthal — two compounds with proven anti-inflammatory powers.

- Green tea. Research from the University of Michigan suggests a mighty compound found in green tea, called EGCG, combats RA inflammation.

- Dark chocolate. Eat small amounts of this in place of junk food. Junk food may cause inflammation, but dark chocolate antioxidants fight to stop it.

Little-known cause of painful joints

Rheumatoid arthritis (RA) may not be the cause of your problems if your joint pain comes with symptoms like bloating, diarrhea, gas, stomach pain, weight loss, and fatigue. Instead, you may have celiac disease. On average, people with celiac disease have symptoms for over a decade before they're diagnosed. If you have celiac disease, you have an allergy to a common food ingredient — gluten. Foods that contain gluten include grains like wheat, rye, and barley, as well as processed meats, pasta, and sauces. Your doctor can test you for celiac disease. If you test positive, a gluten-free diet may ease your symptoms.

Oddly enough, a similar diet may help if you have RA but not celiac disease. Cutting gluten out of your diet and going vegetarian can dramatically cut your risk of heart attack and stroke. That's good news for RA sufferers who have an increased risk for these life-threatening conditions.

In a Swedish study, participants with RA ate either a well-balanced, regular diet or a gluten-free vegetarian diet of fruits, nuts, sunflower seeds, buckwheat, corn, rice, sesame milk, millet, and vegetables — including root vegetables. After one year, those eating the gluten-free, vegetarian diet not only lowered their cholesterol and BMI (body mass index), they also raised their levels of an antibody linked to better heart and blood vessel health.

If you'd like to try a gluten-free or gluten-free vegetarian diet, get advice from your doctor about what to eat and whether you need vitamin and mineral supplements to get all the nutrition you need.

The juice-lover's way to battle RA

Fight inflammation and you may fight rheumatoid arthritis, too. Drinking just 6 ounces of pomegranate juice may be enough to have anti-inflammatory effects in your body, researchers from Case Western Reserve University in Ohio say. Animal research suggests pomegranate juice may lessen the severity of RA.

In fact, one study found that animals given pomegranate juice took significantly longer to get RA than animals that didn't drink the juice. Although more research needs to be done, why not drink pomegranate juice in place of another sweet drink. It can't hurt — and it might help.

Popular sweetener boosts gout risk

Gulp down a sugar-laden soft drink and you just told your body to start producing uric acid. Too much uric acid and you're well on your way to a painful bout of gout. Canadian researchers discovered that drinking just two soft drinks a day increases your risk of developing gout by 85 percent — especially if you're a man. What's more, men who drink only five soft drinks a week still have a 29 percent higher risk than men who don't consume soft drinks.

Not surprisingly, diet soft drinks don't raise your risk. The reason for the difference may be the main sweetener used to sweeten nondiet soft drinks. The sugar typically found in nondiet soft drinks — high fructose corn syrup — puts extra fructose into your body. This extra fructose makes your body produce more uric acid, a known trigger for gout.

Soft drinks aren't the only threat to your health. The Canadian study also found that fructose-rich fruit juices, such as orange juice and apple juice, raise your odds of developing gout. This doesn't mean you should never eat an orange or apple again. But the fewer fructose-laden drinks you have, the lower your risk of gout.

Other natural remedies

Glucosamine and chondroitin — what the headlines don't tell you

The newspapers may proclaim glucosamine and chondroitin don't work, but you might want to take a closer look. According to recent research, some glucosamine supplements work far better than others, and chondroitin supplements still show surprising promise.

Glucosamine. Glucosamine comes in two versions, and it pays to check which one you're getting. When scientists from Nebraska's Creighton University reviewed glucosamine research, they discovered that glucosamine sulfate can help reduce knee pain and slow the progression of knee osteoarthritis (OA). Study results for glucosamine hydrochloride showed it offered no more benefit than a placebo.

Experts say the reason glucosamine sulfate may help your knee arthritis is because it may actually restore damaged cartilage — something no other medication does. In fact, glucosamine occurs naturally in the cartilage of your joints. It helps lubricate joints and prompts cells to rebuild cartilage. Animal research suggests that glucosamine supplements can add extra glucosamine to your joints.

Although glucosamine sulfate may help your knees, it may not work as well for arthritic hips. Two years of daily glucosamine sulfate failed to ease the pain and stiffness in people with early hip arthritis, a Dutch study reported. But more research is needed. After reanalyzing the study, two experts say some details in the study results suggest glucosamine may have more potential to help people with late-stage hip arthritis than early arthritis.

Chondroitin. A recent review of studies found that adding chondroitin to a glucosamine supplement does not make the supplement any more effective. But in Europe, a chondroitin supplement is approved as a prescription drug for arthritis symptoms. What's more, a new study of this product recently found that two years of daily chondroitin not only reduced cartilage loss but also relieved pain faster than a placebo. With such conflicting results among studies, more research may still be needed to determine whether chondroitin helps arthritis sufferers.

Get the most from this dynamic duo. If you'd like to try glucosamine or chondroitin, keep these points in mind.

- Experts recommend taking 1,500 milligrams (mg) of glu-cosamine and 1,200 mg of chondroitin daily.

- For best results, choose pills with a smaller dose — such as 500 mg glucosamine and 400 mg chondroitin — and take the smaller doses throughout the day. Results may take anywhere from a few weeks to several months to show up.

- These supplements may not help people who have extremely severe osteoarthritis.

- Talk with your doctor and pharmacist before trying these sup-plements, especially if you take other medications or have other health conditions in addition to OA.

Simple step prevents disability

Break a hip and there's a 50-50 chance you'll end up in a nursing home. Fortunately, you can cut your risk of fracture dramatically by doing one simple thing — get more vitamin D. It's called the sunshine vitamin because your skin can make it with just a little sunlight. You can also get vitamin D from food, like fortified milk, eggs, and sardines, or supplements. In spite of that, up to 90 per-cent of older adults don't get enough vitamin D. Even worse, one study reports that low levels of vitamin D can boost a woman's risk of fracture by more than 70 percent.

This amazing vitamin can make a difference in your fracture risk because it strongly affects your bones. A lack of vitamin D cripples your ability to absorb calcium and lowers the amount of calcium circulating in your body. This raises your levels of parathyroid hor-mone, which quickly triggers more bone loss. As a result, your danger of osteoporosis and hip fractures shoots up. But here's the good news. Getting enough vitamin D has been linked to less frac-ture risk in older adults.

Find out whether you're getting enough vitamin D and then get more if you need it. To start, ask your doctor if you need the "25 hydroxy D" test to determine whether you're deficient in vitamin D. You're more likely to benefit from the test if you're an older adult because your skin has less ability to make vitamin D than when you were younger. You may also benefit from this test if you have osteoporosis or are at high risk for osteoporosis. Your doctor can help you determine whether the test is worthwhile.

Because your need for vitamin D is likely to go up as you get older, it also pays to find out just how much vitamin D you should be getting every day. The National Osteoporosis Foundation suggests 400 to 800 international units (IU) of vitamin D for people age 50 and under and 800 to 1,000 IU starting at age 51. Other experts recommend 1,000 IU a day to prevent hip fractures. Ask your doctor how much vitamin D you should get. For more information about vitamin D, see "Beat disease with the sunshine vitamin" on page 82 in *Cardio health: fit for life*.

What insiders know about bone-building supplements

Get more bang from your supplement buck with professional secrets from the experts.

Choose the right calcium. Tums, a popular antacid, is a good source of calcium because it's made from calcium carbonate. But if your stomach acid levels are too low, you can't absorb calcium carbonate very well. That's why you should take Tums or other calcium carbonate supplements with meals. Food boosts your stomach acid levels. If you regularly take acid blockers, like Zantac or Prilosec for heartburn, or if you take your supplements between meals, choose calcium citrate supplements. When your stomach acid levels are low, you can absorb more calcium from calcium citrate supplements than from calcium carbonate.

Take your calcium in smaller doses. Your body absorbs the most calcium when you take doses of 500 milligrams (mg) or less at a time. What's more, some experts say that taking several calcium doses of 200 mg or less throughout the day can help preserve your bones.

Beware of drug interactions. Talk to your doctor or pharmacist about how calcium supplements affect prescription drugs you take. These supplements can interfere with some antibiotics, as well as drugs like levothyroxine or bisphosphonates. As if that's not enough, other drugs, like steroids, interfere with calcium. Your doctor or pharmacist can tell you how to deal with these problems.

Read food labels. Tally up how much calcium you get each day from food. Subtract that number from 1,200 mg, or the amount recommended by your doctor, to get the amount you need from supplements. If you already eat plenty of dairy foods or other high-calcium foods, you'll need less calcium from pills.

Get enough vitamin D. In the worst cases of vitamin D deficiency, your body may only absorb 15 percent of the calcium you take in. This matters because your body loses its ability to absorb calcium as you grow older. By age 65, a woman can only absorb half as much calcium as she did during her teenage years. That makes vitamin D even more essential as you grow older. Check whether the vitamin D in your supplement is ergocalciferol (vitamin D2) or cholecalciferol (vitamin D3). Vitamin D3 may be better at raising your vitamin D levels.

Be a wise consumer. Independent testing by Consumer Lab suggests that most calcium and calcium-D supplements contain just as much calcium and vitamin D as they promise on their labels. To make sure you've found a good supplement, look for the CL Seal or the USP-verified symbol on the label.

Easy answer to low back pain

That aching pain in your lower back might be easier to fix than you think. While it's true back pain is a symptom of osteoporosis, sometimes the pain is caused by a different problem — osteomalacia or "soft bone" disease. When you have osteomalacia, your body can't make bone properly so your bones become soft. This condition is less common than osteoporosis, and it can be cured.

The only way to check for osteomalacia is to see your doctor. Depending on what he finds during your exam, he may order a blood test to check your vitamin D levels, a bone density scan, or X-rays.

Certain medications and conditions, such as kidney disease, may cause osteomalacia, but a major cause is vitamin D deficiency. Most important, if you get osteomalacia from too little vitamin D, a combination of vitamin D, calcium, and phosphorus supplements may be all you need to recover within six months.

Beat arthritis pain naturally

Imagine a natural remedy for arthritis pain that works as well as aspirin, ibuprofen, and celecoxib (Celebrex). Studies suggest SAM-e supplements may do just that. S-adenosylmethionine (SAM-e) is a compound your body makes and uses in many vital chemical processes. But if you've been looking for relief from arthritis symptoms, here's why you may want to try SAM-e supplements.

Beats inflammation. SAMe wields anti-inflammatory powers against arthritis.

Repairs cartilage. Thinning and damaged joint cartilage causes your osteoarthritis (OA) symptoms. You'll be glad to know studies suggest SAMe can increase the thickness of joint cartilage, raise the number of cartilage cells, and prevent the cartilage cell damage that may cause OA symptoms.

Zaps pain. SAMe has repeatedly proven better at zapping arthritis pain than a placebo in scientific studies. Researchers discovered that SAMe may be just as good a painkiller as the NSAIDs (nonsteroidal anti-inflammatory drugs) aspirin, ibuprofen, and celecoxib after a month or two of use. Even better, some of those studies suggest that SAMe users may have less risk of miserable digestive side effects than people who use NSAID painkillers.

If you'd like to try SAMe supplements for your OA pain, keep these points in mind.

■ Get your doctor's permission before you try SAMe if you have diabetes because it may lower your blood sugar. If he approves, monitor your blood sugar closely. Your doctor may need to adjust your medication dose to keep your blood sugar from dropping too low.

■ Take no more than 200 milligrams (mg) on the first day and then gradually work up to 800 mg daily. However, be sure to spread out the doses during the day and take no more than 200 mg at a time.

■ Watch out for drug interactions. It may not be safe to take SAMe with some drugs, such as tramadol (Ultram,) meperidine (Demerol,) or antidepressants. It also may not be safe for people with bipolar disorder. Check with your doctor and pharmacist before using it.

- Shop wisely. SAMe doesn't keep well. In some cases, it can break down so quickly you may get less active ingredient than the label shows. To avoid this, buy SAMe in blister packs and look for the more shelf-stable version of SAMe called butanedisulfonate.

- Choose enteric-coated tablets and take them with meals. SAMe may cause unpleasant side effects, like nausea and upset stomach, in some people.

- Compare prices. SAMe can be expensive and insurance doesn't cover it. Check your local GNC and other stores or shop online — *www.vitacost.com* (800-793-2601), *www.swansonvitamins.com* (800-824-4491), and *www.vitaminshoppe.com* (800-223-1216). If you find a good price online, don't forget to figure in shipping costs and check for possible sales tax.

- Be patient. SAMe may take up to eight weeks to relieve your pain, inflammation, and joint stiffness. Plan accordingly.

New way to cut your losses

L-carnitine, a naturally occurring amino acid, can battle bone loss, a preliminary animal study suggests. While there is no recommended dosage for this use of L-carnitine, the Linus Pauling Institute reports that supplement doses usually range between 500 mg and 2,000 mg. Talk with your doctor to learn more about this exciting amino acid.

Why you need more vitamin K

The experts were wrong. Good bone mineral density alone isn't enough to protect you from a hip fracture. Fortunately, vitamin K may go beyond bone mineral density to protect your bones in different ways.

■ Encourages your body to produce more collagen. This extra collagen makes your bones more flexible so they bend a little instead of breaking — like trees swaying in the wind.

■ Stimulates a protein called osteocalcin. Some studies suggest vitamin K play a role in osteocalcin formation. As new bone is created, osteocalcin acts as a quality control manager and makes sure new bone gets woven into a pattern that helps resist fractures.

■ Thickens bone. One study even suggests the right kind of vitamin K can thicken the neck of your femur, the bone that extends from your hip to your knee. Thicker bones may be more likely to foil a fracture.

That's three ways vitamin K may cut your danger of fractures without improving your bone mineral density (BMD). But the vitamin K you know may not be all you need to get the job done.

Meet the new kid on the block. You're probably already familiar with regular vitamin K, the kind you get from dark green, leafy veggies, including spinach, kale, lettuce, and broccoli. Scientists call this vitamin K1 or phylloquinone. But vitamin K1 has a silent partner called vitamin K2 or menaquinone. Some forms of this vitamin are found in meat, cheese, egg yolks, and a fermented soy product called natto. But here's where things get interesting. Your body uses vitamin K1 to make a particular form of vitamin K2 called menaquinone-4 or MK-4. Research suggests MK-4 may do a much better job of getting into your bones than vitamin K1.

Get the scoop. Just because MK-4 shows up in bone doesn't mean it strengthens bone, so Dutch scientists put it to the test. They studied 325 women who did not have osteoporosis. Half the women took 45 milligrams (mg) of MK-4 supplements every day, while the other half took a placebo. After three years, the placebo group had clearly lost bone strength in their hips, but the MK-4 group lost almost none — even though both groups had similar BMD scores. What's more, the MK-4 group scored better on key measures of hip bone strength, including resistance to impact and bending strength, the qualities that make a hip harder to fracture.

Improve your odds. Research shows that people who are low in vitamin K1 are more prone to both low BMD and fractures. Before you take supplements, make sure you eat plenty of dark green, leafy veggies and other foods rich in vitamin K1. Also get plenty of calcium, vitamin D, and exercise to shore up your BMD.

But for maximum protection, talk to your doctor about your risk of osteoporosis and fractures and get his advice on whether you should try vitamin K2 supplements. These supplements aren't safe for everyone. People taking blood thinning drugs, like warfarin, may not be able to take vitamin K supplements without serious side effects. If your doctor approves, take your MK-4 supplements in divided doses, such as 15 mg three times daily. This helps keep your vitamin K levels constant so your bones get uninterrupted protection against disabling hip fractures.

Control arthritis pain with herbs

Herbs like willow bark were helping fight the agony of arthritis long before aspirin came along. While herbal remedies might not be effective for everyone, studies suggest they can significantly ease pain for some people — and you might be one of them.

White willow bark. Studies show that willow bark, the natural version of aspirin, can help fight chronic osteoarthritis (OA) pain. Experts recommend buying a willow bark extract that contains a daily dose of 240 milligrams (mg) of salicin, a compound that acts like aspirin in your body. Be aware that willow bark can cause stomach upset, ulcers, and bleeding in your digestive tract — just like aspirin.

Rose hips. Five milligrams of rose hip powder daily may help diminish OA pain and reduce the need for painkillers, several studies suggest. One study even found that rose hip powder decreases C-reactive protein, a sign of inflammation in your body.

Pycnogenol. Another promising weapon against arthritis is pycnogenol, an extract from the bark of the French maritime pine. In a study of arthritis sufferers, the researchers compared people who took 100 mg of pycnogenol daily to those who took a placebo. After three months, the pycnogenol group reported less pain and stiffness than the placebo group. They were also able to cut back on their painkillers and could walk farther without pain.

Researchers think the anti-inflammatory powers of pycnogenol may help muffle arthritis symptoms. Pycnogenol may also lower blood sugar levels and increase your risk of bleeding, so check with your doctor before you buy it. To avoid possible side effects, take pycnogenol with food.

Boswellia. *Boswellia serrata*, India's version of frankincense, may fight two enzymes that cause your arthritis symptoms. People with osteoarthritis who took 100 mg or 250 mg of enriched *boswellia* extract daily not only reduced their arthritis pain, they also cut their levels of an enzyme that causes cartilage destruction.

The extract was enriched with 3-O-acetyl-11-keto-beta-boswellic acid, the most active compound in *boswellia*. That compound may help squelch a second enzyme that promotes inflammation, a key cause of your symptoms. A word of caution — *boswellia* may aggravate gastroesophageal reflux disease (GERD) and gastritis.

Before trying herbal products, check with your doctor. Some of these items — especially rose hips, willow bark, and *boswellia* — may interact with medications you already take.

Bring RA to its knees

Rheumatoid arthritis (RA) may be tough on your joints, but an herbal compound, known as borage, may be even tougher on RA. This herb grows around the Mediterranean and the Middle East. Its seeds contain a fatty acid called gamma linolenic acid (GLA) that fights inflammation.

One study found that people who took 1.4 grams a day of GLA in borage seed oil reduced both the number and the severity of their tender and swollen joints in just six months. If you'd like to try borage oil, talk to your doctor. If she gives you the green light, read bottle labels carefully to find the amount of GLA different brands contain. Recommended amounts for RA range from 360 milligrams to 3 grams.

Healthful living

10 secrets to make life with arthritis easier

Arthritis can make the daily tasks of living tough, but you can make them simple again with these tips.

■ Stop struggling with the lid on the mayo jar. Buy a squeeze bottle of mayonnaise instead. Squeeze bottles of jelly, mustard, and other condiments may help as well.

■ Get a better grip on your car steering wheel. Purchase a pair of weight-lifting gloves from your local discount store.

■ Solve a handbag problem. If sore fingers or a sore shoulder makes carrying a purse too painful, buy a small backpack. Tuck your purse inside the backpack or use the backpack as your new purse.

■ Make your bed more easily. Trade your current wrinkle-prone bedspread for a light comforter. Then, instead of pulling and adjusting the sheets and bedspread to smooth every little bump, just pull the comforter over the sheets and your bed is made.

■ Go easy on your trigger finger. If squeezing the trigger on a spray antiperspirant hurts, switch to a stick or roll-on antiperspirant.

■ Do tough tasks less often, preferably on days when you feel better. For example, don't just cook one night's dinner. Cook enough for several nights and freeze the food you're not ready to eat. If a container is hard to open, buy the economy size. Open it only once — to empty its contents into easy-to-open containers.

■ End the gas cap blues. Use a round, rubber jar opener or a pair of rubber gloves to open your gas cap more easily.

■ Lighten up. If heavy drinking glasses are hard to handle, switch to hard, plastic glasses — like the ones kids use.

■ Tame tough lids. For pop-top and peel-here containers, use a butter knife, letter opener, or metal fingernail file to help open them.

■ Ditch the dish towel. If drying with a dish towel hurts your hands, dry your dishes on a rack instead.

Healing moves for arthritis sufferers

Ease your arthritis pain with gentle activities like walking, water exercise classes, and tai chi. This "therapy in motion" may even help you avoid hip and knee replacement surgery.

Consider the findings. The Arthritis Foundation Exercise Program is low-impact, gentle exercise you can do while sitting or standing. After just eight weeks of this program, people with osteoarthritis (OA) reported less pain and fatigue, more strength, and they were able to do everyday tasks easier, a recent study reports. Those who continued the program beyond eight weeks also experienced less stiffness. To learn more about this program and how to find it in your area, see the following story, "Discover no-sweat pain relief."

If you prefer something simpler, consider walking. People who walk for at least 30 minutes five or more days a week may lower their levels of C-reactive protein and other compounds linked with inflammation, which triggers arthritis symptoms.

Check out the rewards. Depending on the exercise you do and how often you do it, you may find yourself losing weight. Moreover, if you're overweight, those vanishing pounds may help cut your risk of a hip or knee replacement down the road.

A study of nearly 40,000 Australians found that those who weighed the most or had the highest body mass indexes (BMIs) were at least three times as likely to have a hip or knee replacement as people who weighed the least or had the lowest BMIs. This may happen for two reasons.

■ Extra weight puts an extra load on your joints, which worsens arthritis and destroys your cartilage even faster than it normally would. The more quickly arthritis breaks down your cartilage, the more likely you are to need joint replacement surgery.

- Some fat cells don't just sit quietly. They pump out inflammatory compounds. Some of these compounds are famous for destroying the cartilage in your joints.

Combine physical activity with a sensible, reduced-calorie diet and you may shed pounds, ease the load on your joints, and prevent the flood of inflammatory compounds from fat cells. That may be enough to help you avoid joint replacement surgery when you're older.

Take the next step. If you're ready to find out what getting active can do for you, get your doctor's permission first. If she says yes, get her advice on which kinds of activities are safe and effective for you. Your answer may be as simple as a 10-minute walk three times a day, or you may get the chance to try new options, like tai chi or water exercise classes.

Discover no-sweat pain relief

You may think the slow, gentle motions of tai chi look too easy to be good for you. But this ancient form of exercise has been used for centuries to keep those of advanced years feeling young and happy, and now it's available to seniors everywhere.

The benefits. Tai chi can improve your mobility, breath control, and relaxation — even if you have arthritis. In fact, tai chi may be particularly good for you if you have arthritis, Texas Tech University researchers say. They asked older adults with knee arthritis to try six weeks of tai chi classes, followed by six weeks of home tai chi training. By the end of their training, study participants had less knee pain and the knee pain they did have was less severe. Their ability to do everyday tasks improved, too. But these benefits disappeared after six weeks without tai chi. If you try tai chi, continue to do it regularly.

Who can do tai chi. You don't have to be in good health or great shape to do tai chi. You simply follow a pattern of flowing movements through various poses and stances. The motions are slow and gentle so you don't need strong muscles or super flexibility. You never fully extend or bend your already-tender joints. In spite of that, studies suggest tai chi can make your muscles stronger. Tai chi may also improve your flexibility and balance, reduce stress, and lower your risk of falls. And if you're worried about osteoporosis, you'll be glad to know tai chi may help prevent bone loss in women who are past menopause. On top of all that, the breathing techniques often included in tai chi may promote breath control and relaxation.

Before you begin. Nearly everyone can do tai chi without danger, but play it safe and ask your doctor's permission first. While you're at it, ask if he can recommend any tai chi classes particularly suited to people with arthritis. If he can't, try these options.

- Check the local senior center or the YMCA.

- Call or visit *www.arthritis.org* (800-283-7800) to find out if the Arthritis Foundation's Exercise Program is available near you.

- Visit *www.taichinetwork.org* to find schools and teachers in your area.

- Ask friends and family to recommend a class or instructor.

When you find a class, ask the instructor if you can observe a session before you sign up. Some types of tai chi are more strenuous and complicated than others, so watch first to see if this class has what you need.

Remember, too, the people in the study practiced tai chi for 12 weeks to ease their arthritis. For best results, commit to at least 12 weeks of classes.

Soothe achy joints with water

Most people try to "stay out of hot water," but if you've got arthritis, getting into soothing warm water may dowse your arthritis pain. Water's natural buoyancy eases the weight-bearing strain and impact of activities like walking by 50 to 90 percent. That's why you may move more easily in water than on land.

What's more, water exercise may help you even more than regular exercise. A study from Brazil's Federal University found that people with arthritis who did exercises in water for several months experienced a bigger decrease in pain than people who did similar exercises on land.

Work out your pain. Your doctor or physical therapist may give you specific water exercises to do on your own. But if that's not the case, consider these intriguing options.

- Try the Arthritis Foundation Aquatic Program. Call 800-283-7800 or visit *www.arthritis.org* to find classes near you. You may be charged a small fee for each class, so ask about cost before you sign up. Because the goal of this program is to safely and harmlessly improve your range of motion, the exercises are mostly gentle bends and stretches.

- For a more intense workout, consider water aerobic classes at your local fitness center or YMCA.

Soak away discomfort. If taking a class doesn't work out, try a good soak instead. A Turkish study found that people who took 20-minute soaks in 98-degree Fahrenheit water twice daily for 10 days reduced their pain more than people who just took pain relievers. But to protect your heart from danger and still get results, some experts recommend soaking in water that's only 92 to 96 degrees.

Find relief with mineral springs. If you ever find yourself in a spa town like Hot Springs, Ark., or at a resort that offers a mineral spa, give it a try. Hungarian researchers found that people with osteoarthritis who soaked 30 minutes daily in warm mineral waters containing fluoride, sodium bicarbonate, and metaboric acid needed fewer painkillers after just three weeks. Maybe your spa won't contain the same minerals, but a joint-soothing soak in any warm water may be beneficial — and you may enjoy the experience.

Dirty little secret eases soreness

Hot mud may cool your arthritis pain, just like hot water. Turkish scientists asked people with knee osteoarthritis to try regular 30-minute applications of hot mudpacks on their knees. Half the group used mudpacks cushioned by a nylon shield, while the other half placed the hot mudpack directly on their knees. Both groups had less pain after the mud-packs, but the group that applied the mudpacks directly on their knees got the most relief. Researchers think compounds in the mud may offer added protection from pain.

Many spas offer mud baths with a specially mixed combination of peat and mineral-enriched clay. If you get the opportunity, try a mud bath or mud treatment, and you might discover a new way to ease your hurt.

Stop the ache without dangerous drugs

You used to be stuck between a rock and a hard place — either take NSAID pills and endure the unpleasant side effects or live with a whole lot of pain. But now you have a third choice — topical creams. Check out these pain-relieving ingredients in some over-the-counter creams.

NSAIDs. Topical NSAID creams are just as effective as NSAID pills, reports the Federal Agency for Healthcare Research and Quality. And unlike NSAIDS you take by mouth, these creams are less likely to cause side effects like indigestion, higher blood pressure, and asthma flare-ups.

Salicylate. Creams that contain pain-relieving salicylate, a cousin to aspirin, are readily available. Aspercreme and Myoflex are just two of the many choices.

Capsaicin. You can send your pain packing with creams containing capsaicin, an ingredient derived from hot peppers. These creams can relieve your aching joints without serious side effects. Capsaicin works by depleting substance P, a protein-like compound that transmits pain impulses to your brain. Capsaicin can cause a warm, stinging, or burning sensation, but regular use will cause the sensation to fade in a few days.

Menthol. You can also try products that contain menthol, a peppermint plant compound with pain-fighting powers.

If over-the-counter creams aren't enough, ask your doctor about stronger prescription products, like Voltaren gel or the Flector patch. Creams can be a powerful part of your pain protection arsenal, but they won't always be your best choice. They can cause side effects such as skin rashes. And they do their best work if you only have a small area where you're having pain. For widespread pain, pain-relieving pills may still be your best bet.

Put the brakes on arthritis

Using a cane may help prevent knee arthritis from getting worse. An Australian study found that people who used canes reduced the stress on one of their knees. But to take advantage of this, you must choose the right cane and use it correctly.

When buying a cane, ask the salesperson about either a center balance cane, which is popular with people who have arthritis, or a quad cane, a good choice for people who need maximum weight-bearing support. The right size cane will reach your wrist anytime you bend your arm enough to place your hand at hip level.

To use the cane correctly — say to protect your right knee — hold the cane with your left hand. Then without moving your arm away from your body, use your wrist to shift the bottom end of the cane forward as you move your right foot forward. As you put weight on your right foot, use the cane to help bear your weight and make sure your right foot never supports your weight without help from the cane. The Australian researchers found this reduces the strain on your right knee. To protect the left knee, hold the cane in your right hand and use it to help your left foot support your weight.

Cheap protection for knees and hips

Going barefoot may be better for your knees and hips than wearing expensive shoes designed for comfort and support. Computerized analysis of 75 people found that walking barefoot put less strain on knees and hips than walking in shoes.

But those cute and fun flip-flops everyone is wearing are not all bad. While long-term use may give some people foot problems, they can actually be better for your knees than some expensive shoes. Just be sure to look for flip-flops with the American Podiatric Medical Association's Seal of Acceptance.

---

6 simple steps to foil foot pain

You don't have to live with painful feet. The solution may be as simple as switching shoes or getting the right shoe insert. Soothe your soles, tame toe pain, and help your heels with these tips.

- Leave wiggle room. To prevent corns and calluses and to stop making hammertoes and bunions worse, choose shoes with enough room to wiggle your toes.

- Get measured. If you haven't had your feet measured in years, do it now. Feet get longer and flatter as you age. Your current shoes may be up to two sizes too small.

- Ditch the heels. High heels help cause hammertoes, bunions, heel pain, corns, calluses, toe cramps, and more. If you must wear heels, stick with the ones that are 2 inches high or less.

- Rotate your shoes. Toe cramps happen because your shoes repeatedly put too much pressure on the same part of your foot. Ease that pressure by rotating among flats and shoes of varying heel heights.

- Seek support. If you have flat feet, your feet may lean inward — or over-pronate — as you walk. Choose shoes that support your arch and heel or seek out shoe inserts that support your feet or promise to prevent over-pronation.

- Soothe your arches. Select shoes that leave plenty of room for your feet if you have high arches. Also, look for gel inserts or soles with soft padding.

Insoles and inserts can increase your comfort. You can buy two types — over the counter and custom-made "orthotics," which a doctor tailors to your feet. A review of studies found that custom orthotics can help relieve pain in people with rheumatoid arthritis, highly arched feet, or unusually prominent big toe joints — in a matter of months. If you wear an insole or insert that's not right for your particular problem, you could make your feet worse.

According to the American Academy of Orthopedic Surgeons, these are the kinds of inserts and insoles routinely recommended for common foot problems.

Foot problem	Recommended item
bunions	bunion shield pad
flat foot pain	semi-rigid insert, long arch pad, inner heel wedge, or extended heel counter
hammer toe	toe crest pad
plantar fasciitis	prefabricated heel insert

Medical alternatives

Help for hurting knees

Take a shot at arthritis pain relief with an amazing new treatment that works by restoring a desperately needed compound to your knee joints. Best of all, your poor knees could feel better for months.

Discover what's missing. Hyaluronic acid (HA) occurs naturally in the cartilage of your knee joints. Because HA acts as a lubricant and shock absorber, it cushions the ends of your thigh bone and lower leg bone near your knee joints. This helps them move smoothly without ever banging into one another. HA may also battle arthritis more directly by fighting pain and inflammation.

Studies suggest some people with osteoarthritis have below-normal levels of HA in their knees. If you can imagine how a car would run with too little lubricating oil and worn-out shock absorbers, you can see how too little HA is bad news for your knees. In fact, just a half-teaspoon of missing HA may literally leave you knee deep in pain.

Fortunately, three to five weekly HA injections in your doctor's office may make a big difference. According to researchers, these shots can give six months of pain relief to at least 90 percent of those with mild or moderate knee arthritis. Some people have gotten up to 18 months of relief.

What to expect. If you'd like to try HA injections, keep these things in mind and talk them over with your doctor.

- Effectiveness. These injections are about as effective as NSAIDs (nonsteroidal anti-inflammatory drugs, like aspirin or ibuprofen) or corticosteroid injections when given to men, but they may give women less relief.

- Side effects. The shots have few serious side effects, but some people may experience milder effects, like temporary swelling, itching, or pain near the injection site.

- Cost. They're expensive, so make sure your health insurance or Medicare plan covers these injections.

Lasting RA pain relief on the horizon

Imagine a future where you are free of rheumatoid arthritis (RA) pain. Researchers are working on two injections that may help that dream come true.

Vaccine. Your immune system protects your body by fighting infection. But if you have an autoimmune disease, like rheumatoid arthritis, your immune system goes haywire and attacks your joint tissues.

According to preliminary research, scientists can use a sample of your white blood cells to create special "tolerogenic dendritic" cells. These cells order your immune system to "stand down" instead of attacking your tissues. A vaccine of these cells injected into your joints may squelch your RA symptoms. Scientists are currently testing this vaccine on humans for the first time, so stay tuned.

Gene therapy. Just four weeks after treatment, two women with advanced RA reported less pain and swelling in joints injected with a gene that inhibits a protein called interleukin-1, a key villain behind the breakdown of cartilage in RA. In fact, one woman found that pain in the treated joint had vanished completely. Although more testing is needed, scientists hope to make this shot available as early as 2013.

What you should know before arthritis surgery

Be well-informed before you decide to have hip or knee surgery for arthritis. And make a list of questions for your doctor as you consider your choices.

Surprising news about arthroscopic knee surgery. During arthroscopic surgery, the doctor cleans out bone and cartilage fragments that can cause pain. However, a study of people with moderate to severe osteoarthritis of the knee found that those who had arthroscopic knee surgery showed no more improvement in pain, stiffness, or quality of life than people who had nonsurgical treatments.

If you'd like to avoid surgery, aim for a nonsurgical treatment plan similar to the one used in the study. This plan included physical therapy, exercise, pain relievers and anti-inflammatory drugs, hyaluronic acid injections, glucosamine supplements, and lessons about managing arthritis.

But surgery isn't always a poor choice. According to the *Journal of Family Practice*, you may still benefit from arthroscopic surgery if you have a large tear in your meniscus — an arc-shaped stretch of cartilage that protects your knee.

Learn the latest about joint replacement. Although surgery should usually be a last resort, that may not be true for joint replacement surgeries, like knee and hip replacement. Some experts say that people who delay surgery until arthritis makes them severely disabled never recover as fully as those who have the surgery earlier.

Besides, joint replacement surgery has a high, long-term success rate. It may also help relieve pain and improve your quality of life — especially if you're an older adult who hasn't gotten relief from other arthritis treatments.

Know your options. Here are a few other common surgery options for people with arthritis along with key points you should know about each one.

osteotomy	<ul><li>removes damaged tissue and reshapes bone deformed by that tissue</li><li>eases symptoms</li><li>used when only part of the knee is damaged</li><li>best for adults with above-average weight who are under 60 years old</li></ul>
unicompart-mental knee arthroplasty	<ul><li>for joint damage restricted to one side of the knee</li><li>uses small implants instead of full joint replacement so you keep more knee ligaments and freedom of movement</li><li>recommended for sedentary, but not obese, people age 60 or older</li></ul>

autologous cartilage implant	• replaces damaged cartilage with healthy cartilage from another part of your knee • best for people age 40 and younger
hip resurfacing	• alternative to hip replacement that preserves more bone • serious complications — like fractures below the neck of the femur, or thigh bone — after surgery is more likely in people over age 55 and women of all ages

Say good-bye to osteopenia drugs

You've been diagnosed with osteopenia — the first step toward osteoporosis — and you've tried to get ahead of the game by taking osteoporosis drugs. But now, guidelines from the National Osteoporosis Foundation (NOF) suggest that some women with osteopenia may not need these drugs.

The purpose of osteoporosis drugs is to prevent disabling fractures. Yet, osteopenia by itself doesn't guarantee you're at high risk for a fracture. In fact, the latest NOF guidelines say your doctor shouldn't prescribe osteoporosis drugs for osteopenia unless you meet two requirements:

■ You were diagnosed with osteopenia based on a bone scan.

■ You have at least a 3 percent risk of fracturing a hip or a 20 percent risk of any major osteoporosis-related fracture within 10 years.

Doctors can estimate your risk of these fractures using a new online tool called FRAX from the World Health Organization. Combined with the new NOF guidelines, your FRAX results may keep you from taking bone-building medications you don't need.

And there are good reasons to avoid taking these drugs if they're not necessary. Recent research has discovered three rare — but dangerous — drug side effects you should know about.

Severe pain. Call your doctor if you experience severe joint, muscle, or bone pain after starting on alendronate (Fosamax), risedronate (Actonel), pamidronate (Aredia), ibandronate (Boniva), etidronate (Didronel), tiludronate (Skelid), or zoledronic acid (Reclast or Zometa). This pain may be temporary, or it may mean you should switch to a different drug.

Thigh fracture. A type of thigh bone fracture usually associated with car accidents has begun showing up in people who take bisphosphonate drugs, like Fosamax, Actonel, or Boniva. Even worse, these fractures occurred while people were standing, strolling, or doing other activities that cause no major impact trauma to thigh bones. Researchers are investigating whether osteoporosis drugs may be responsible for this rare — but alarming — side effect.

Jawbone decay. A new study suggests that osteonecrosis of the jaw, a rare disorder that causes destruction of the jawbone, may occur following dental work in up to 4 percent of people who take Fosamax.

You can help keep your bones strong by doing a few simple things. Get enough calcium and vitamin D every day, limit your alcohol consumption, and don't smoke — whether you have osteopenia or not. Also, aim for regular doses of weight-bearing activity, such as walking, as well as exercises that strengthen your muscles.

If you take medication for osteopenia, talk to your doctor about the new NOF guidelines and ask whether you can safely stop taking the drug. Your doctor can also tell you more about possible side effects of your medication and what you can do about them.

Little-known way to treat a common disorder

Early treatment of a common genetic disorder could add years to your life. Otherwise, this condition can cause arthritis, heart disease, impotence, depression, and damage to your pancreas that can lead to diabetes.

The disorder is named hemochromatosis and five out of every 1,000 white people are at risk of developing it. Often the result of faulty genes, hemochromatosis causes your body to absorb too much iron. The extra iron can build up in your heart, liver, and pancreas and cause them to fail. Fortunately, an easy and inexpensive treatment can bring those iron levels back down. It's called phlebotomy, and it's just like donating blood.

Hemachromatosis screening isn't necessary for everyone. The National Institutes of Health suggests doctors consider screening anyone who has one or more of the following — heart disease, diabetes, impotence, elevated liver enzymes, severe and lasting fatigue, arthritis, or a relative with hemochromatosis.

An aspirin a day keeps osteoporosis away

That baby aspirin you take every day may not just be good for your heart. It might help keep your bones strong, too. After taking low-dose aspirin every day for three months, mice prone to osteoporosis improved their bone density. Some studies suggest aspirin works the same way in humans as in mice.

If that's true, aspirin may prevent your immune system from accidentally attacking the stem cells that later turn into bone-making cells. If more of those stem cells survive, you'll end up with more bone-making cells and better bone density. But more research is needed.

If you already take aspirin for your heart, your bones may be reaping the benefits. However, if you don't take aspirin every day — at least 75 milligrams (mg) to 100 mg — check with your doctor before you try it. Aspirin can cause stomach bleeding, and it can be dangerous when taken with some prescription drugs.

When bone scans come up short

Nearly 50 percent of the women who had a fracture after age 50 did not have osteoporosis, as defined by current bone mineral density (BMD) test guidelines. Their bones were simply too strong. That's why experts now suspect BMD tests only supply part of the information needed to predict your risk of fractures.

BMD tests only measure how much bone you have, but physical traits, medications you are taking, family history, health conditions, and personal habits, like drinking alcohol and smoking, also determine how well your bones resist a fracture.

Beware hidden fracture danger

Two groups of people — men and people who have congestive heart failure — are at higher risk for a disabling hip fracture than they realize. Here's what you need to know to take steps to protect yourself and beat the odds.

Only 12 percent of men age 50 and older have osteoporosis now, but the American College of Physicians (ACP) expects that number to grow 50 percent by 2024. Even worse, fracture rates are likely to double by 2040. To prevent this, the ACP has issued new screening guidelines to help men avoid both osteoporosis and fractures.

These guidelines recommend your doctor determine your risk of fracture by the time you reach age 65. Examples of factors that raise your fracture risk include low body weight, smoking, not getting enough calcium, lack of physical activity, and previous fractures from weak bones. If your doctor thinks you have a high risk of fracture, the ACP recommends a bone scan to check for osteoporosis.

Although health experts aren't sure why, people who have congestive heart failure have at least six times more risk of hip fracture and four times more danger of any fracture compared with people who have had heart attacks or other heart conditions.

If you're a man over age 50 or if you've ever had congestive heart failure, ask your doctor about your fracture risk and how you can protect yourself. Your doctor will assess your odds and recommend nutrients, lifestyle changes, and possibly medications to lower your fracture risk.

New hope for stubborn heel pain

Your plantar fasciitis pain hasn't gotten better even though you've spent a year doing stretches, wearing arch supports, and following your doctor's instructions. It's time to consider new options like these.

Percutaneous ultrasound guided approach. After other treatments fail, your doctor may suggest an option called shockwave therapy. Unfortunately, it's very painful. That's why Italian scientists tested another treatment called "percutaneous ultrasound guided approach" (PUGA). The scientists gave PUGA to 44 people who had tried regular medical treatment for plantar fasciitis but didn't get any relief. Three weeks later, the pain and symptoms had disappeared in 95 percent of the study participants. Even better, this treatment is quicker, cheaper, and less painful than shockwave therapy. Here's how PUGA works.

A radiologist injects local anesthesia right where it hurts. You need to be numb because needle punctures are crucial to this treatment. According to the Italian scientists, needle punctures in just the right places create bleeding that helps heal your plantar fasciitis. The radiologist uses ultrasound equipment to pinpoint exactly where the needle punctures will do the most good. He makes the punctures with an empty needle and then injects the area with a steroid to fight inflammation and pain. That's all there is to it.

Botox. Small studies suggest Botox injections into the foot can relieve pain and improve walking ability. But more research is needed to prove the effectiveness and safety of this treatment. Talk to your doctor to learn the latest news about this treatment.

Secrets to speedy digestion & supercharged metabolism

Start with breakfast for slim waistline

Fewer people eat breakfast today than they used to, but if you want to lose weight you need to buck the trend. Lots of research links skipping breakfast with obesity. Calories count, but trying to save them for later in the day could backfire.

■ People who regularly ate breakfast in one study did eat more calories every day, but they gained less weight with age than breakfast-skippers. What's more, eating breakfast for six weeks helped people lose more weight than eating a large dinner.

■ Breakfast-eaters who do lose weight are actually better at keeping it off.

■ People who eat more calories in the evening see a bigger rise in their body mass index over time, a measurement of obesity. Obese women, on the other hand, tend to eat fewer calories in the morning than lean women.

At this point, experts know that eating breakfast helps you maintain a healthy weight, but some foods are better at it than others. We're not talking grapefruit and celery, either. Foods like oatmeal, eggs, high-fiber cereal, milk, and even Canadian bacon practically force your body to lose weight. You can make these delicious foods part of your morning routine and know they're doing your body good.

Natural aid to weight loss

A calcium deficiency could be driving you to overeat. Researchers think the brain can tell when you're running low on this vital mineral. It compensates by pushing you to eat more food, a phenomenon called "calcium appetite."

Unfortunately, it's easy to get too little calcium when you start cutting calories, and calcium appetite can sabotage your efforts. Eating more dairy may help squash hunger and your desire to eat. Studies suggest dairy calcium may control weight better than supplements.

50-cent meal clobbers weight and cholesterol

Beginning your day with a hearty breakfast can help you lose weight, but make it a bowl of oatmeal and you'll lower your cholesterol, too. It just goes to show, some of the healthiest foods are actually the cheapest.

Oatmeal, along with many cold cereals, is packed with insoluble fiber that can turbo-charge your diet. People who ate the high-fiber cereal Fiber One for breakfast felt fuller and ate fewer calories the rest of the day compared to people chowing on a low-fiber cereal like Kellogg's Cornflakes. That's significant, because Fiber One actually has fewer calories.

A larger study had similar results. Out of nearly 18,000 men, those who ate breakfast cereal of any type consistently weighed less — and they were less likely to become overweight with age if they ate at least one serving of cereal daily. Oatmeal may be an even better bet, since study after study shows oat bran can cut both total and "bad" LDL cholesterol. Spice it up with cinnamon or add variety with slices of seasonal fruit.

Lose the belly, not your bones

Boosting your daily dairy protects your bones while dieting and may even aid your weight-loss plan.

Bone up on protection. Losing weight can help plenty of health problems, but it also tends to cause bone loss and boost your fracture risk. High-protein diets may be especially harmful, because the more protein you eat, the more calcium you lose through urine — calcium that may be coming from your bones.

New research shows high-protein diets don't have to rob your bones, if you eat plenty of dairy while you're on them. During the course of one year, dieters followed either a high-carb diet with two daily servings of dairy, or a high-protein diet with three. The three-serving diet boosted calcium intake and prevented people from losing bone while they lost weight.

Slim down and stay that way. Keeping the weight off is almost as hard as losing it in the first place. Don't worry about dairy sabotaging your trim figure. Although dairy foods may add calories to your diet, they can also keep you from feeling hungry. Folks who ate three servings of dairy daily may have eaten more calories than people who only got one serving a day, but they didn't gain weight.

Casein, a protein in dairy, delays stomach emptying, so you feel full longer. Out of two diet plans — one heavy on the casein and one not — the high-casein diet suppressed hunger 41 percent more, boosted satiety by one-third, kept blood sugar and insulin levels from spiking after meals, and made people burn more calories. In the long-run, casein may even trim fat.

Focus on low-fat. The trick is to get more dairy without adding saturated fat, which you can do by focusing on low-fat milk, yogurt, and cheeses. Start your morning with a high-fiber cereal swimming in skim or low-fat milk, or enjoy a cup of low-fat yogurt alongside your oatmeal.

Egg-ceptional way to shed pounds

Sticking to a diet is hard, but choosing eggs over bagels in the morning can make it a lot easier. Men who had an egg breakfast ate fewer calories the rest of the day, had more stable blood sugar levels, and were more satisfied and less hungry three hours later than guys who ate a bagel.

What's surprising is that the two meals contained the same number of calories. The difference — bagels are big on carbohydrates but low in protein and fat. Eggs are just the opposite, and they could help you control your weight while dieting.

Eating two eggs for breakfast five days a week for eight weeks, while also cutting their daily calories, helped overweight dieters lose 65 percent more weight, shrink their waistlines one-third more, shed 16 percent more body fat, and feel more energetic than dieters who ate a bagel breakfast, even though they got the same amount of calories every day. However, cutting calories was still important. People who didn't but still ate eggs did not drop weight.

Eggs didn't seem to raise people's cholesterol or triglyceride levels in this study, either. In fact, experts think their natural cholesterol may actually boost your levels of "good" HDL cholesterol. They're also rich sources of an antioxidant called lutein, which helps put a lid on inflammation. Chronic inflammation contributes to hardening of the arteries and insulin resistance, which can lead to metabolic syndrome as well as predict the development of heart disease.

If the studies bear out, eggs may help you head off these conditions and maintain a healthy weight. Talk to your doctor first before making them a regular part of your morning routine, especially if you're trying to cut your cholesterol intake.

Eggs and diabetes: a dangerous combination

You can eat an egg every day and not increase your risk of stroke or heart attack — unless you have diabetes. In the famous Physician's Health Study, people with diabetes saw their risk of dying rise with eating just one egg a week. Eating seven or more eggs a week doubled their mortality rate. Plus, eggs seemed to increase their risk of heart attack and stroke.

The same wasn't true for people without diabetes. They had to eat at least seven eggs a week before their mortality risk went up, and even then it only rose 22 percent.

Experts aren't sure what accounts for this difference, but, in the meantime, eat eggs sparingly if you suffer from diabetes.

Melt away fat with lean protein

A slice of Canadian bacon alongside those morning eggs can help you feel full longer, which in turn could help you eat less the rest of the day. Protein makes you feel more sated after meals than carbohydrates or fat, so you're not tempted to snack as much or overeat later. Modestly upping your protein intake while cutting calories may help you lose fat, develop more lean muscle, and keep the weight off after finishing a diet.

In fact, higher-protein diets may be better for shedding pounds and keeping them off than either carbohydrate- or fat-focused diets. In a new study, two groups of obese people lost weight and tried to keep it off. Those sticking to a low-fat, high-protein diet kept off the pounds better over three months than those on a low-fat, high-carb diet. The protein-eaters even continued to shed flab, despite eating as much food as they wanted.

Protein forces your body to burn more calories than other nutrients in two ways.

- You burn 65 to 75 percent of your energy during rest, and the more muscle you have, the more energy you burn. Protein boosts lean muscle mass, helping you burn more calories even while resting.

- Your body can't store extra protein the way it can extra fat. The body has to deal with it right then. All this added work burns more energy than normal.

Breakfast is by far the best time to build in protein. Eating it at breakfast is more filling and satisfying than eating protein later in the day, at lunch or dinner.

You don't have to go to extremes, though. Moderate amounts may be enough. Some experts worry about the long-term safety and health effects of high-protein diets, and moderate- and high-protein diets have similar benefits on insulin sensitivity and your ratio of fat to muscle.

Aim to meet at least the Recommended Dietary Allowance (RDA) for protein. That's about 55 grams (g) for a 150-pound person, or 80 g for a 220-pound person. Otherwise, you might not get enough to rev up your weight loss. If you're feeling ambitious, try to meet the moderate-protein goal of getting one-fourth, or 25 percent, of your daily calories from protein.

Trim the fat from high-protein diets

The wrong high-protein foods can actually contribute to insulin resistance, a forerunner to diabetes.

Protein is made up of amino acids, and up to one-fourth of them are branched-chain amino acids (BCAAs). Meat protein, in particular, is packed with BCAAs, and that can be a problem.

BCAAs by themselves don't seem to cause a problem. But when eaten along with lots of fat, these compounds may contribute to insulin resistance. If you're on a high-protein diet, be sure to choose lean protein, and cut back on fatty foods in general.

Calories the key to trimmer figure

Cut your calories to drop the weight quick and keep it off. Limiting calories is the #1 change you should make to your diet, according to the latest research.

A new study shows it's not which diet you follow, but how many calories you eat, that counts. People followed one of four eating plans and were offered weight-loss counseling. Diets were either low or high in fat, average or high in protein, or low or high in carbohydrates, but they did have one thing in common — they all trimmed 750 calories a day out of the people's normal diet.

Surprisingly, everyone lost about the same amount of weight, as well as improved their cholesterol and insulin levels, during the two-year study. Turns out, what they ate didn't matter. How many calories they ate did. So did the support they received from weight-loss counseling. Those who attended were more likely to slim down, shedding about half a pound for each session.

Experts now say any calorie-cutting diet can be successful if it doesn't go too strongly against your preferences — a low-carb diet will be tough to sustain if you love carbohydrates — and if you approach it with enthusiasm and stick-to-it persistence.

5 incredible weight-loss secrets

Losing weight is as much about what you do eat as what you don't. Some foods virtually melt away fat, while others pack it on. Follow these easy eating tips to start shedding weight fast.

Sip some green tea. If it works for mice, it might work for you. Mice with a fat gene who got the human equivalent of seven cups of green tea daily gained 25 percent less weight, were less likely to develop fatty liver disease, and enjoyed lower cholesterol and triglycerides than mice without green tea.

Scientists say catechins, special compounds in the soothing drink, seem to keep your body from absorbing and storing fat. At the same time, they may prompt you to burn more fat for energy.

Indulge in dark chocolate. Thank the Dutch. A Danish study found dark chocolate makes you feel more sated than milk chocolate. Young men who ate the dark treats ate 15 percent fewer calories when they sat down to an all-you-can-eat pizza buffet two and one-half hours later, compared to those who ate milk choco-late. So when you crave sweet, go dark.

Aim for more arginine. Your body uses arginine to make nitric oxide, and together they help burn fat and prevent it from being stored. Rats given arginine as part of their diet gained less fat, partic-ularly belly fat, than regular rats. Arginine did, however, beef up their muscles. Experts think this natural compound affects how your body uses energy, building muscle with it rather than storing it as fat.

The body naturally makes this amino acid, but you can get it from food, too. Canned light tuna, tilapia, spinach, roasted pumpkin seeds, walnuts, raisins, and chicken breast are all good sources.

Try a few chili peppers. Capsaicin, the spicy compound in hot peppers, squashes the growth of fat cells and even kills them. Rats fed high-fat diets laced with capsaicin didn't gain weight, whereas those without it did. It may also guard against obesity-related inflammation and complications, such as hardening of the arteries and diabetes. Who knows, you just may discover a love for cayenne, banana peppers, and jalapeños.

Hold the MSG. It's often added to processed, prepackaged foods for flavor, but a Chinese study found the more MSG people eat, the more likely they are to be overweight. In fact, people who used the most were nearly three times as likely to be overweight as those using the least. Experts say the seasoning may damage the part of the brain that controls appetite and affect your hormones in ways that contribute to obesity.

Surprising source of weight gain

Those diet sodas may secretly be sabotaging your weight-loss plan. Here's how experts think it works. In childhood, your body learns that sweet-tasting foods contain more calories. To avoid overeating, it begins using sweetness to gauge how many calories it has eaten.

Artificial sweeteners like aspartame, saccharin, sucralose, and ace-sulfame K may confuse your body, since foods made with them taste sweet but pack fewer calories. As the theory goes, your body learns it can't rely on its sweet sense to judge calorie content. As a result, it starts thinking that all sweet foods have few calories, even those sweetened with sugar, and that it can eat as much as it wants.

That has been the case in animal studies. Compared to rats fed sugar-sweetened food, those getting saccharin-sweetened food ate more calories, gained more weight, packed on more body fat, and didn't compensate for eating sweet stuff by cutting back on calories elsewhere, as they normally would.

Not all experts agree on this link, but they do agree that consciously counting calories along with exercising is a proven way to control your weight.

Drop 5 pounds without breaking a sweat

A glass of water before meals may not be as good as soup at helping you cut calories, but it still fights flab. One study found that drinking water in place of other beverages helped women on diets lose an extra five pounds a year. They also shrank their waistlines and shed fat, and all of it regardless of the type of diet they were following.

Secret to losing weight without dieting

Drinking a glass of water before dinner may not help you lose weight, but eating that water in a tasty soup before dinner will. And in one study, drinking water alongside a casserole wasn't as filling as a soup containing the same ingredients. That's because liquids you drink don't satisfy hunger as well as liquids you eat.

Think of it as a mind trick. Your brain perceives the beverage as satisfying thirst, not hunger. Plus, pure liquids leave the stomach faster than soupy ones, which may explain why a watery food fills you up better than a drink.

Eating a bowl of soup before the main course can help you cut calories without making you feel like you're on a diet. Case in point — people who ate soup before an entrée ate less total food and 20 percent fewer calories at one meal. And past research shows that enjoying soup regularly for several months cuts calories, leaves people feeling fuller, and helps them shed pounds.

If you can't stand soup, there's still hope. It's just one of many foods that do the same thing. The secret is energy density — how many calories a food has per ounce (or portion). Foods that take up a lot of space on your plate but have few calories, like broth-based soups, have low energy density. Those that pack a lot of calories in a small portion, like cheesecake, have high energy density. Piling your plate with low energy-dense foods will help you feel full while adding fewer calories — a sure recipe for shedding fat.

What makes a food less energy-dense? Generally, having lots of water or fiber. Both add bulk and weight but few or no calories. Fruits, veggies, low-fat milk, cooked grains, fish, and poultry generally have high water contents. So do soups, stews, casseroles, and fruit-based desserts. Many are also high in fiber, a dieting double whammy.

By focusing on low energy-dense foods, you'll eat more food but fewer calories and less fat, not to mention get more disease-fighting vitamins and minerals every day.

Follow their lead. People on low energy-dense diets tend to eat more fruits and vegetables, focus on low-fat dairy, and avoid exclusionary diets, like Atkins. Instead, they get to enjoy food from every food group. They do, however, limit red meat, sweetened cereals, and soft drinks.

Eat more, not less. Simply adding water- and fiber-rich veggies to your regular casserole can slash its energy density, with no need for a special recipe. Tossing in broccoli, celery, or carrots lets you put the same amount of food on your plate for fewer calories, or eat more food for the same calories. Try replacing some of the pasta in dishes and salads with vegetables, too, and slash the calories by 30 percent.

Substitute smartly. Beef up casseroles and entrées with mushrooms instead of meat. People who ate the same lunch made with beef one day then mushrooms the next consumed the same amount of food but a whopping 420 more calories at the beef lunch. Substituting mushrooms didn't affect the food's tastiness or people's sense of fullness.

Eye the ingredients. Fat boosts the energy density of foods. It packs more than twice as many calories per ounce as carbohydrates or protein. When evaluating a new recipe, check the amounts of fatty ingredients, like butter or oil, it calls for to get an idea of how energy-dense it will be.

Fill up with fewer calories

Keep in mind that not all fruits are low energy-dense. Dried ones like raisins contain little water. And while 100 calories worth of grapes will fill almost two cups, 100 calories worth of raisins fills a measly one-fourth cup. This means grapes will fill you up with fewer calories.

Warning: sweetener may sabotage weight loss

Check your drinks and packaged foods, and you'll find high-fructose corn syrup (HFCS) listed more often than not. Recent news stories say HFCS is safe, but don't believe it yet. Most of these have been released by the Corn Refiner's Association, the industry that makes this sweetener.

The latest research still shows plenty of cause for concern, suggesting HFCS leads to weight gain and more belly fat, and may boost your risk for heart disease and diabetes. Here are some of its possible pitfalls.

Increases your appetite. Fructose and glucose, two types of sugar, affect your brain and appetite differently.

■ Fructose makes you want to eat more, boosting your chance of becoming obese.

■ Glucose makes you feel full and eat less.

That poses a problem, since more manufacturers have switched to sweetening food and drinks with the fructose-based corn syrup.

Fattens you up. Your body naturally turns some sugar into fat. In people who drank a beverage containing fructose or glucose, their bodies turned more sugar into fat and did it faster when that sugar was fructose, rather than glucose. "Our study shows for the first time the surprising speed with which humans make body fat from fructose," said lead researcher Dr. Elizabeth Parks, associate professor of clinical nutrition at the University of Texas Southwestern Medical Center.

What's more, their bodies continued storing more energy as fat after the fructose drinks than after the glucose ones, proving that once you start the process of fat synthesis from fructose, it's hard to slow it down, she said. The process may be even worse in overweight people because their metabolism is already off.

Hikes heart disease risk. In a telling new study from the University of California-Davis, overweight people who drank beverages sweetened with fructose saw a bigger rise in their triglycerides and "bad" LDL cholesterol than people drinking glucose-sweetened drinks.

And although both groups gained about the same amount of weight during the study, the fructose-drinkers put on more belly fat. Put these changes together, and you may end up with a higher risk of heart disease.

The bottom line, though, is that while high-fructose corn syrup may not be healthy, it's not the only problem. "There are lots of people out there who want to demonize fructose as the cause of the obesity epidemic. I think it may be a contributor, but it's not the only problem," said Parks. "Americans are eating too many calories for their activity level. We're overeating fat; we're overeating protein; and we're overeating all sugars."

Still, she recommends limiting foods that contain added fructose, such as those made with high-fructose corn syrup. Foods that naturally contain fructose, like fruits, don't pose a danger. Experts say these pantry staples are the biggest sources of HFCS for most people:

- sweetened sodas, fruit drinks, and sports drinks

- desserts

- breads, including bagels, tortillas, biscuits, and muffins

- ready-to-eat cereals

Simple solution to staying slim

Eating more whole-grain foods can help you keep that youthful figure. The USDA's Dietary Guidelines for Americans now say eating three or more servings of whole grains daily can help keep your weight under control, and a new study found women who eat one or more servings of whole grains daily have slimmer waistlines and are 60 percent less likely to be overweight.

Unfortunately, only one out of 10 women in this study met their goal of three servings daily. Almost half ate none at all. They must not have known what they were missing.

Thanks to this healthy habit, women who ate whole grains also got more fiber; vitamins A, E, and B6; and more calcium, iron, folate, and magnesium. Other studies show whole grains can keep you from gaining weight over time, too.

Findings like this are good news for more than just your vanity — waist measurements and your waist-to-hip ratio strongly predict disease risk in overweight people.

Whole grains have a vital role to play. They're an excellent source of fiber, which can make you feel fuller and more satisfied. Building high-fiber foods into your diet, in turn, can help you eat fewer calories and control your weight.

"Whole-grain foods" means exactly what you'd think. They are made using the entire seed (kernel) from the grain. Processing, or refining, grains and turning them into foods can strip away parts of the seed — the healthiest parts, like the bran and germ. Aside from fiber, whole grains usually pack much more calcium, magnesium, and potassium than refined grains.

These foods aren't hard to find, either. Oatmeal, brown rice, and popcorn are natural whole-grain foods. So are corn on the cob, wild rice, buckwheat, cracked wheat (bulgur), and quinoa, among others.

Try replacing some of the refined grains you eat, like white rice, white bread, and regular pasta with their whole-grain counterparts. Aim to make at least half the grains you eat whole grains. It's a quick and easy way to stay nutritionally fit and physically trim as you age.

Fight fat: feast on summer fruits

A fresh fruit cocktail is just what the doctor ordered if you're trying to banish that belly. Colorful cherries, berries, and grapes are naturally sweet, low-calorie snacks packed with plant compounds that help melt away fat.

Try a different cherry. Similar to tart cherries, Cornelian cherries are traditionally used to treat diabetes in China, but these natural wonders can promote weight loss, lower cholesterol, improve insulin levels, and heal fatty livers — even while on a high-fat diet. That's the case for mice, at least, according to a study out of Michigan State University. Cornelian cherries are chock full of natural compounds, called anthocyanins, with the potential to prevent obesity and battle high blood sugar.

Benefit from blueberries. Anthocyanins are the same compounds that give plants and fruits their blue, purple, and red colors. As you might imagine, berries are especially rich in them. In fact, blueberries alone boast 21 different anthocyanins.

Blueberries prevented weight gain and belly fat buildup in an animal study in part by changing the genes that affect how the body processes fat and sugar. Experts say changes like these could improve insulin sensitivity and prevent fat gain. They may also help you feel full and eat less.

Not all research agrees, though. In one study, eating blueberries in addition to a high-fat diet led to both weight and fat gain in mice. But there are two sure ways to make them work for you — munch on them fresh or frozen in place of potato chips when you need a snack, and top off oatmeal and cereal with them instead of sugar.

Eat the whole grape. Whatever you do, don't spit out the seeds of Chardonnay grapes. They're packed with powerful antioxidants called polyphenols. Scientists put two groups of hamsters on high-fat diets but added grape seed extract for one group. Those not getting the extract gained belly fat, developed insulin resistance, and had high blood sugar and triglycerides.

Hamsters getting grape seeds didn't suffer from the same changes. What's more, they had 45 percent lower levels of the hunger-causing hormone leptin, but 61 percent higher levels of the hormone adiponectin, which can help trim body fat.

Even dried grapes are good for weight loss. Both raisins and walking lowered men and women's "bad" LDL cholesterol in one study, but raisin eaters got an added boost, as the tiny fruits also squashed hunger.

Fruit packs weight-loss punch

Fruit juice just doesn't pack the same health punch as a piece of fruit for weight loss and diabetes prevention.

Women who added three more servings of whole fruit to their normal daily diets slashed their risk of type 2 diabetes 18 percent. Drinking fruit juice, however, canceled out those gains. Having just one more glass of juice a day actually increased their type-2 risk by 18 percent, perhaps because of the loads of sugar in many juices.

Similarly, people who ate a whole apple before a meal consumed 187 fewer calories than people who drank apple juice. Both the apple and the juice packed the same calories and fiber, so scientists know those weren't the cause. Instead, they have two theories:

- People felt fuller after eating the fruit because they expect food, but not liquids, to fill them up.

- Whole fruit takes more chewing than processed versions of it, including applesauce or juice. The act of chewing may make you feel full and eat less.

So grab an apple or pear before your next meal, and limit the sugary fruit juices you drink.

Low-fat dairy cuts diabetes risk

Milk really does do your body good, especially if you're at high risk for type 2 diabetes. Dairy's unique combination of magnesium, calcium, and vitamin D poses a triple threat to this debilitating disease.

Make way for this mineral. A look at seven studies found that people with diabetes tended to have less magnesium in their blood than healthy folks. All in all, every 100-milligram (mg) increase in magnesium levels slashed their risk another 15 percent.

The mineral probably improves insulin sensitivity, since low magnesium levels are linked to insulin resistance, glucose intolerance, and high insulin levels. Luckily, getting more of this mineral improved insulin sensitivity in one study, although the benefit topped out at 325 mg of magnesium daily.

Only magnesium from animal or dairy sources slashed diabetes risk in a Chinese study, though. Eating vegetables rich in it did not. Experts suspect the vitamin D that often accompanies magnesium in meat and dairy products may boost your body's absorption of it. Plus, cooking veggies may sap their stores of this mighty mineral.

Bone up on vitamin D and calcium. The amounts of vitamin D and calcium you get may have a huge impact on whether you develop diabetes. Both nutrients may help regulate glucose tolerance, insulin sensitivity, and inflammation, plus play a role in keeping pancreatic beta cells working, the cells that make insulin.

Getting at least 1,200 mg of calcium along with at least 800 IU (International Units) of vitamin D each day cut type 2 risk by one-third in one study, while women who got the most calcium every day cut their risk by one-fourth. When researchers tested vitamin D levels in 808 people, those with the least were much more likely to show signs of insulin resistance.

To ward off diabetes, some experts recommend getting 1,200 mg of calcium and 1,000 IU of vitamin D daily. Unfortunately, most people over age 70 fall far short of those goals, averaging only 500 to 700 mg of calcium daily, while up to half of adults in the United States may have a vitamin D deficiency. In fact, some experts think vitamin D and calcium deficiencies are partly to blame for the explosion of diabetes in this country. After all, the same groups that tend to be D-deficient — seniors, obese people, sedentary people, and minorities — are also more likely to develop diabetes.

While most dairy products are packed with calcium, only fortified dairy foods like milk contain vitamin D. Yogurt, cheese, and ice cream often don't, which means getting this much D from dairy alone can be a challenge, as shown in the table on page 184.

Salmon, tuna, and mackerel are other excellent sources, but even then, some people may have trouble getting enough vitamin D from food.

Older adults, in particular, should talk to their doctors about whether they need vitamin D, and even calcium, supplements. In any case, the National Institutes of Health warns against getting more than 2,000 IU of vitamin D daily. More can be toxic.

Dairy food	Calcium (mg)	Vitamin D (IU)
skim milk, 1 cup	306	100
mozzarella cheese, part-skim, 1 oz	219	0
Swiss cheese, 1 slice	221	12.3
Yoplait Original yogurt, 6 oz	200	80
Dannon Light & Fit yogurt, 6 oz	150	80
Yoplait Thick and Creamy yogurt, 6 oz	300	80
Dannon Activia, plain, 8 oz	450	0

Nuts take a bite out of diabetes

They're the latest food on the front lines in the war against diabetes. Walnuts, almonds, and peanuts are part of a nutty solution to deal with this disease. That's because they're packed with polyunsaturated fatty acids (PUFAs), healthy fats known for helping your heart, liver, and now diabetes.

Pack in the prevention. In the Nurse's Health Study, women who ate nuts five or more times a week dropped their diabetes risk by

27 percent. Even peanut butter protected, cutting the risk 21 percent in women who ate it more than five times weekly.

Get insulin under control. Walnuts are another top-notch source. Overweight people with diabetes who ate about 1 ounce daily for a year not only got more PUFAs naturally than non-eaters, they also slashed their fasting insulin levels in the first three months. Enjoying a sprinkling of nuts alongside carbohydrate-filled foods can also cap the rise in blood sugar after meals if you already have type 2.

Ward off complications. PUFAs may help prevent age-related mental decline, a particular danger for people with type 2 diabetes. Experts tracked nearly 1,500 women over age 70 who had type 2. Those with a history of either loading up on trans and saturated fats or eating too few PUFAs were much more likely to suffer mental decline with age.

Perhaps more worrisome, tests showed the minds of women who had eaten the most "bad" fat seemed to be seven years older than those of women who had eaten the least trans fat during their lifetime. Cutting back saturated and trans fats and eating more polyunsaturated fats may prevent this downward slide. That's not all.

■ Walnuts also pack a potent second punch, since they're a great source of a special PUFA called omega-3. This fatty acid seems to squash inflammation, a major culprit in complications caused by diabetes.

■ Nuts help block heart disease as well. People with diabetes face three to four times the risk of heart disease as average people. Besides that, nuts contain very little carbohydrate, making them perfect for low-carb diets.

Keep in mind, not all nuts are this good for you. Some, like almonds, walnuts, and hazelnuts, are rich in healthy, unsaturated fats. Others, such as cashews, macadamias, and Brazil nuts have hefty doses of saturated fat.

Banish cravings with MUFAs

A slice of avocado, a dash of olive oil, or a handful of nuts with your lunch could help you eat less the rest of the day. These foods are full of monounsaturated fat (MUFA), and new research shows a particular MUFA called oleic acid can help calm hunger.

Oleic acid prompts the small intestine to produce the hunger-fighting compound oleoylethanolamide (OEA). In turn, OEA trips the switch that makes your digestive tract tell your brain it's full. The result — you feel fuller, longer, which can help stop snack cravings between meals.

Reel in protection from deadly diseases

The healthy fats in fish provide a one-two punch to both diabetes and colon cancer risk.

Scale down diabetes risks. Cultures that eat loads of fish, like Alaskan Eskimos and folks in Greenland, have historically low rates of diabetes. Eskimos who eat the most fish are also the least likely to develop glucose intolerance.

The secret weapon — a special polyunsaturated fat named omega-3. Feasting on foods rich in it may help prevent and even reverse insulin resistance. Compared to healthy people, those with insulin resistance have much more saturated fat and much less polyunsaturated fat in their bloodstream. Simply picking different foods can change that and improve your insulin sensitivity.

Omega-3s can help you dodge diabetes complications, too. These fishy fats cut triglycerides in half in people with diabetes, a boon for heart health, and other studies suggest they may ward off diabetic nerve, kidney, and eye diseases.

Cut the line on colon cancer. Supping on one to two servings of fish a week sliced colon cancer risk a clean 30 percent in an Eastern European study. Serving it up even more often slashed the risk almost in half. Eating meat, on the other hand, upped the cancer risk. The Physician's Health Study found similar results. Men who ate the most fish — a little over six servings each week — had 40 percent less chance of developing colon cancer.

Fish are the biggest source of omega-3s in your diet, and these scrappy fats seem to protect against colon cancer in lab and animal studies. Indeed, men who got the most omega-3s, regardless of how much fish they ate, still had less chance of getting this disease. Here's why.

■ Omega-3s may help quench inflammation that can lead to colon cancer. Plus, they may keep cancer cells from multiplying and trigger them to die.

■ Fish are also full of other cancer-fighting nutrients, like vitamin D.

■ Fitting more fish into your diet may mean you eat less meat, further reducing your colon cancer risk.

For the most omega-3, think fatty, dark-meat fish like salmon, or canned light tuna, pollock, and catfish, all of which tend to have low mercury levels. The American Dietetic Association suggests eating two servings of fish a week.

Cut carbs to control diabetes

Counting carbohydrates is a lot easier than following the glycemic index (GI), and it may help control diabetes better than insulin injections and without dangerous episodes of low blood sugar.

Doctors who treat people with type 2 diabetes report good success rates using low-carb diets. In some cases, people can eventually come off their diabetes medications, saving themselves money along with the other benefits.

Cutting back on carbohydrates seems to improve blood sugar control and reduce ups and downs in your insulin levels. It's as good as low-fat diets for weight loss, and it may help prevent diabetes in people who have metabolic syndrome.

The American Diabetes Association (ADA) recommends carb counting as a good way to control your blood sugar. In fact, the amount of carbohydrate in a food predicts how it will affect your blood sugar better than the glycemic index does. A food's GI does impact blood sugar, but the ADA suggests focusing first on some sort of carb counting. Then, if you want or need to, you can fine-tune your blood sugar control further with the glycemic index. Visit the Web site *www.glycemicindex.com* for a searchable list of food GIs.

Spotting carbohydrate content is simple. Read the food label on packaged foods to find out how many grams of total carbs each serving contains. Remember to check the serving size, and make sure you eat that amount. Bigger servings mean more carbs.

For fresh foods, you'll have to estimate. The ADA says these food portions each pack about 15 grams of carbohydrate. A low-carb diet should limit carbs to either 130 grams or 26 percent of your daily calories.

- small piece of fresh fruit

- slice of bread or 6-inch tortilla

- one-half cup of oatmeal

- one-third cup of pasta or rice

- one-half cup of black beans or a starchy vegetable

- one-quarter of a large baked potato

- two-thirds cup of plain, fat-free yogurt

- one-half cup of a casserole

- one cup of soup

Low-carb diets may not be right for everyone, so check with your doctor before making major changes in what you eat. Even if you decide to give it a try, have your doctor keep a close eye on your blood sugar. She may need to lower the dosage of your diabetes medicine before you begin the diet.

Kick cancer with low-GI foods

Sticking to a low-GI diet can do more than manage diabetes. It could also keep thyroid, colon, and endometrial cancers at bay.

The glycemic index (GI) measures the effect a food has on your blood sugar. High-GI foods raise blood sugar more than foods with a medium or low GI value. In an Italian study, people who ate mostly high-GI foods were up to 70 percent more likely to develop thyroid cancer compared to those on low-GI diets.

Glycemic load (GL) had an even more profound effect on thyroid cancer. The GL takes into account both a food's carb content, minus its fiber, and the portion size. In the same study, people with high-GL eating habits were two to three times more likely to develop thyroid cancer as those who ate mostly low-GL foods. Along the same line, researchers have found a link between high-GI and high-GL foods and colon and endometrial cancers.

After a meal, your digestive system breaks down the carbohydrates into sugars, which get absorbed into your bloodstream. As your blood sugar levels rise, the pancreas releases insulin to help your cells absorb all that sugar. High-GI and high-GL foods cause a bigger rise in blood sugar than low-GI and low-GL foods do. To deal with those spikes, your body releases more insulin.

That's where the cancer risk comes in. High insulin levels have been fingered as a risk factor in several types of cancer. Insulin works like a growth hormone in colon and thyroid cells. It ups the activity of insulin-like growth factor (IGF), which makes cells multiply and keeps them from dying. Insulin can also affect sex hormones such as estrogen, which play a major role in certain cancers.

Insulin may not be the only culprit, however. A diet rich in high-fiber foods may cut your colon cancer risk, and high-fiber foods tend to have lower GI values. The sugar sucrose on the other hand — which increases the GI value of foods — may boost the risk of colon cancer.

Top-notch colon defense

Fresh whole fruits, vegetables, and legumes are on the front lines of colon cancer prevention, and even treatment. These "secret" healing foods are inexpensive and could prevent about a third of all cancer cases. But you probably won't see them advertised as potent cancer-fighters. Since they are whole foods, minimally processed, and easy to grow in your own backyard, manufacturers simply can't make much money off them.

Experts at the National Cancer Institute found that eating foods loaded with natural antioxidants called flavonols made colon cancer up to 90 percent less likely to return. Lab studies show flavonols can stop cancer before it starts by protecting cells against damage and preventing them from mutating. These compounds also seem to keep cancer from growing by quenching inflammation, stifling the spread of cancer, and triggering diseased cells to die.

Fruits and vegetables such as beans, apples, yellow onions, broccoli, kale, and leeks are all excellent sources, but you'll have to make an effort to eat more of them. The average Western diet doesn't provide enough flavonols for real colon cancer protection. Start loading your plate with these inexpensive, top-notch defenders.

Legumes K.O. colon cancer. African American men and women who ate the most dried beans, lentils, and split peas were 80 percent less likely to develop colon cancer. Plus, beans battle breast, prostate, lung, liver, and ovarian cancers. Legumes pose a unique triple-threat because they're:

■ chock-full of fiber. Bean fiber cut the risk more than any other type in a Japanese study.

■ filled with phytochemicals. These plant compounds may protect cells from genetic damage, helping to prevent cancerous changes.

■ crammed with healthy carbs. Your body can't break down the carbohydrates in beans. Instead, they ferment in your colon, churning out anti-cancer compounds while doing so. Pinto, baked, kidney, lima, and navy beans all cut colon cancer risk in studies.

Crucifers crush disease. Besides flavonols, cruciferous vegetables contain other compounds that help can cancer, including sulforaphane and indole-3-carbinol. These compounds help damaged cells die so they don't turn cancerous.

Raw veggies may be the way to go. Men got 30 percent more sulforaphane when they ate their broccoli raw than when they cooked it, plus they absorbed it faster. Crucifers can lose anywhere from 30 to 60 percent of their anti-cancer compounds during cooking. A study on red cabbage, however, found cooking it over low heat on the stove, or on medium in the microwave, actually boosted its cancer-fighting power.

Summer fruits stymie cancer. Extracts made from peaches and plums could be a sweet way to squash colon cancer growth. Polyphenols, potent antioxidants in these two fruits, seem to force cancer cells to mature to the point where they can't reproduce anymore, a cancer cell's version of menopause. Bite into these seasonal fruits for a sweet dose of protection.

Sweet news: some sugars good for diabetes

Natural sugars, including date and dark brown sugars, are packed with antioxidant compounds that may help manage diabetes. The darker, the better. Dark brown sugar, for instance, contains 4,000 more antioxidant compounds than white sugar, gram for gram.

That's important because having high blood sugar produces too many free radicals, compounds that can damage your cells and lead to disease. Antioxidants like those found in dark sugars, however, can quench free radicals before they do harm.

Date sugar, dark brown sugar, and evaporated cane juice also block an enzyme in the intestines that controls how much sugar from food actually enters your blood stream. Blocking this enzyme may prevent dangerous blood sugar spikes after meals.

Bake or sweeten with dark brown sugar in place of white, when possible, and look for date sugar and evaporated cane juice on the ingredient list of food packages.

Turn off stomach pain with sprouts

Broccoli just got better for you. Grazing on the young, tender sprouts may protect against serious digestive ills, including ulcers, gastritis, and stomach cancer.

The nasty bacterium *H. pylori* is often the culprit behind all three problems, and roughly half the people in the world are infected with it. Now, researchers at Johns Hopkins University may have discovered a natural way of nixing it and guarding your gut.

People infected with *H. pylori* ate 2.5 ounces of broccoli sprouts every day for two months. The sprouts didn't totally banish the bacterium, but they did reduce the severity of the infection.

That's crucial, because antibiotics don't always cure an *H. pylori* infection. Some strains of the bacterium have become drug-resistant. Failure to wipe it out leaves many people more vulnerable to stomach cancer, the second-most-common cancer worldwide, and the second-most deadly. Fortunately, broccoli sprouts may help suppress the infection.

Broccoli is crammed with a compound called sulforaphane that works like an antibiotic against *H. pylori*. It triggers cells in your body, especially in your digestive tract, to churn out enzymes that protect your DNA from damaging chemicals, inflammation, and oxidation. For the biggest impact, munch on the sprouts rather than mature florets.

"Broccoli sprouts have a much higher concentration of sulforaphane than mature heads," explains Jed Fahey, a nutritional biochemist at Hopkins and one of the researchers behind the study.

Secret anti-aging agent that does it all

A common spice used by millions may have incredible powers against weight gain, diabetes, Alzheimer's, cancer, indigestion, and even skin problems like psoriasis. Best of all, it's probably in your kitchen right now — and if it's not, it should be.

Turmeric is the yellow ingredient in curry powder, a popular seasoning used in Asian food, medicine, make-up, and dye for more than 2,000 years. Now modern science may have a new use for it.

Immune cells called macrophages live in fat tissue throughout your body, cranking out molecules known as cytokines. These can inflame your heart and pancreas and worsen insulin resistance.

Curcumin, a powerful compound in turmeric, crushes inflammation by squashing the number of macrophages and slowing down their activity. As a result, curcumin could help you dodge diabetes, obesity, and other illnesses linked to runaway inflammation. In a lab study, obese mice that ate it:

■ were less likely to develop insulin resistance and high blood sugar, even if they ate lots of fat.

■ lost weight and body fat, despite being on a high-calorie diet.

■ cut the level of inflammatory compounds at work in their bodies.

■ had higher levels of adiponectin, a hormone that improves insulin sensitivity and protects against inflammation and hardening of the arteries.

Diabetic mice that ate curcumin had lower blood sugar and HbA1c levels (a measure of diabetes control) as well as lower cholesterol and triglycerides. And this ancient spice doesn't stop there.

Clobbers colon cancer. The compounds in curcumin may keep precancerous colon cells from multiplying, plus trigger them to die, in people who have already had colon polyps removed. They may also quiet inflammation by stopping colon cells from producing the inflammatory compound COX-2. Studies show limiting COX-2 can stifle tumor growth and the spread of colon cancer.

Helps you avoid Alzheimer's. Thanks to its antioxidant and anti-inflammatory power, curcumin reduced the buildup of beta-amyloid and brain plaque in lab studies. Add to that, a human study found elderly Asians who ate curry at least occasionally scored better on brain function tests than those who rarely ate it.

Soothes psoriasis. Curcumin may help treat autoimmune diseases such as psoriasis in two ways.

- As a powerful antioxidant, it quenches free radicals in your skin, reduces inflammation, and helps wounds heal faster.

- It may also help regulate your immune system, preventing out-of-control immune responses and inflammation that attack the body.

Eases indigestion. Nine out of 10 people who took curcumin supplements for a week saw their indigestion symptoms at least partially improve. Some felt completely better.

Cools a burning gut. Curcumin may help prevent ulcers when taken alongside medicines that tend to cause stomach and intestinal ulcers. It may even treat ulcerative colitis (UC). It helped maintain remission and prevent relapse in people with this condition who took one gram of curcumin twice a day alongside their regular medicine for UC.

People in India get about one teaspoon of turmeric daily just from food. You can take it as a standardized supplement as well. Still, experts warn that getting small amounts of curcumin from food is best, since the supplements can irritate your stomach at high doses or with long-term use. Straight, store-bought turmeric generally boasts a lot more curcumin than curry powder seasoning.

Add a dash of black pepper to turmeric- or curry-seasoned meals to boost the spice's healing power. Piperine, a natural compound in pepper, boosts your body's absorption of curcumin by 2,000 percent, helping you get more of this very good thing.

Think twice about this spice if you have gallstones or gallbladder disease, though. Turmeric could make your gallbladder contract. Also consider skipping it if you:

- suffer from diabetes or low blood sugar, or if you take drugs to help lower your blood sugar.

- regularly take blood thinners, anti-platelet drugs, aspirin, or nonsteroidal anti-inflammatory drugs like ibuprofen.

- have liver disease, since turmeric may harm the liver in high doses.

Get milk to kick colon cancer

Dairy isn't just for strong bones anymore. Mounting evidence shows the calcium, magnesium, and vitamin D in dairy foods like milk can curb cancerous changes in the colon.

Cancer-proof your colon. Past research has consistently shown that dairy and calcium cut colon cancer risk. In one study, men and women who either got the most calcium or ate the most dairy every day had less chance of developing digestive cancers, especially colon cancer. Men trimmed their risk by 16 percent; women, 23 percent.

Scientists suspect calcium keeps cancer cells from multiplying and triggers them to die, at least in the digestive tract. There, it binds to bile and fats, which may protect the lining of your large intestine.

Make magnesium a priority. Calcium alone may not be enough, however. A recent study found that calcium supplements cut the recurrence of colon polyps, but only if people were also getting enough magnesium in their diets. The ratio of calcium to magnesium could be the key. The more calcium you get, the more magnesium you may need to see a drop in your colon cancer risk.

Make sure you're getting plenty of both from the foods you eat. Start the day with an oat bran or shredded wheat cereal, finish it with a brown rice or spinach dish for dinner, and munch on a handful of almonds or peanuts in between for your daily dose of magnesium.

Vanquish disease with vitamin D. Sunlight reduces the rate of many cancers, but it has the clearest impact on colon cancer. Research as far back as 1941 showed a link between where you live and your chances of getting this disease. For instance, the North, which gets less sunlight during part of the year, has higher rates of colon cancer than the South, where sunlight is plentiful almost year-round. For more info on this topic, see "Beat disease with the sunshine vitamin" on page 82 in *Cardio health: fit for life*.

Researchers recently discovered that people with the highest levels of vitamin D in their blood were half as likely to develop colon cancer as those with the lowest. And for every two cups of milk people drank, they sliced about another 12 percent off their risk. Eating cheese helped, too. For every 8.8 ounces of ricotta cheese they ate each day, their colon cancer risk dropped another 17 percent.

Cells in many parts of your body, including the colon, process vitamin D. In those areas, D may stop cancer cells from multiplying and spreading, and trigger them to die. As with magnesium, calcium may only protect against this disease if you also get plenty of vitamin D.

Can the coffee to control diabetes

Regular coffee may help prevent type 2, but people who already have diabetes should stick to decaf. In one study, people with diabetes who got the equivalent of four cups of coffee had higher blood sugar levels throughout the day, bigger swings in their blood sugar and insulin levels after meals, and overnight episodes of low blood sugar.

Experts think caffeine is the culprit, and it could be secretly sabotaging your efforts to control diabetes. Consider switching to decaf and avoiding other caffeine sources, such as sodas and caffeinated teas.

Morning 'joe' is healthy hero

That daily cup of joe does more than wake you up. It may also guard your gut and ward off diabetes.

Say goodbye to gallstones. Women who drank four to six cups of coffee daily over the course of 20 years were one-fourth less likely to need gallstone-related gallbladder surgery. That translates into many fewer surgeries, since gallbladder surgery is one of the most common operations in the United States.

In fact, most research on coffee and gallstone disease shows a protective effect. Coffee and the compounds in it stimulate the release of a hormone, cholecystokinin, that makes your gallbladder contract. They also prevent the cholesterol in bile from crystallizing into stones. Caffeine alone isn't the cure, though. Experts point to coffee's combination of magnesium, potassium, niacin, insoluble fiber, and antioxidants as the secret to its protection.

Unfortunately, decaf coffee doesn't seem to offer the same protection. The processing used to decaffeinate it may also strip away many of these helpful compounds.

Get the drop on diabetes. Sipping on either regular or decaf may slash your risk of type 2 diabetes by making your body more sensitive to insulin and improving your glucose tolerance.

Once again, caffeine may not be the answer. You should probably thank other coffee compounds, including chlorogenic acid and quinides. Both men and women seem to benefit, and the more coffee you drink, the lower your risk drops. People who enjoyed four or more cups a day were substantially less likely to develop diabetes.

Guard against liver cancer. In a study of more than 60,000 people, the more coffee they drank, the lower their risk of liver cancer. Those who drank two to three cups a day cut their chances by one-third; four to five cups, by almost a half; and six to seven cups, by nearly two-thirds.

Researchers think caffeine, chlorogenic acid, coffee bean antioxidants, and the natural oils in coffee may help keep a lid on high blood sugar. This, in turn, can ward off type 2 diabetes, a disease also linked to liver cancer. Enjoying a morning cup of joe also seems to protect against chronic liver disease and cirrhosis, both of which boost your risk of liver cancer.

Other natural remedies

Zap fat and build muscle faster

One popular dietary supplement really does have anti-aging effects, including reducing dangerous fat around your middle. Conjugated linoleic acid (CLA) is a natural polyunsaturated fatty acid in milk and meat fat, but for slimming down, you can get it from supplements.

People who took CLA for six months in one study lost belly and leg fat, shrunk their waistlines, and even put on muscle. Obese women improved the most, regardless of what they ate or how much (or little) they exercised.

A review of all the studies done on CLA and weight loss found similar results. Overall, CLA helped people lose an extra 0.8 pounds of fat for every four weeks they took it. After six months, however, the effects reached a plateau, and the extra fat-burning edge it gave seemed to wear off.

Pay close attention when shopping for this supplement. It comes in different varieties, some better than others. The safest and most effective one contains two types of CLA — the cis-9, trans-11 isomer and the trans-10, cis-12 isomer. Not all brands list which formula they use. If nothing else, check the ingredient list and make sure it consists of at least 75 percent conjugated linoleic acid.

For fat loss, a dosage of 3 to 4 grams a day worked in some studies, although people in the six-month study took 4 grams, three times a day. You may feel nauseous or have an upset stomach or diarrhea after taking it. Side effects like these tend to go away after a couple of weeks of treatment. In the meantime, try taking the supplement with milk or another protein-filled food.

Put more pep in your step

Get more get-up-and-go regardless of your age by restocking your body's natural stores of L-carnitine. You need this molecule to process energy and turn it into a form your body can use. Unfortunately, your carnitine levels start dropping around age 70. Supplements may help fill the void.

A group of centenarians, ranging from 100 to 106 years old, gave them a try. Those who took 2 grams of L-carnitine daily for six months ended up with less total body fat, more muscle, more physical and mental energy, higher scores on tests of thinking skills, and the ability to walk farther, compared to those getting a fake pill.

---

2 easy ways to rev your metabolism

Make your body work harder without breaking a sweat. Emerging evidence shows two compounds can help you burn more fat while fighting inflammation.

Burn fat faster with CoQ10. Coenzyme Q10 (CoQ10) is a compound your body makes to create energy inside its cells. Unfortunately, you make less of it with age, if you have heart disease, or if you take statin drugs. But you can bump up your levels by taking a supplement.

Healthy men burned more fat while exercising when they took 30 milligrams (mg) of CoQ10 after breakfast than when they didn't. Best of all, they didn't have to work out super-hard to see these results. They simply did a low-intensity workout, spending 10 minutes on a stationary bike.

The supplement may have helped their muscles use oxygen more efficiently. If that's the case, experts suspect CoQ10 could boost the efficiency not just of muscles in your arms and legs, but also your heart and breathing muscles.

Talk to your doctor before trying CoQ10, especially if you have diabetes or take blood thinners or blood pressure medicine. To boost your body's absorption of it, consider buying the softgels rather than hard tablets, and take them with meals.

Treat obesity with resveratrol. This plant compound found in grapes and red wine could help treat obesity. In lab studies, resveratrol stopped fat cells from multiplying, kept young fat cells from maturing into full-fledged ones, and triggered them to die.

By fiddling with fat cells, this compound may help prevent obesity-related diseases such as diabetes and heart problems. That's because fat cells churn out compounds that cause chronic inflammation in your body, which science links directly to these diseases.

Resveratrol may be able to break this cycle by stopping fat cells from producing these inflammatory compounds. It even shows promise in treating diabetes directly through better blood sugar control.

Pairing this natural compound with another one, quercetin, strengthens its fat-fighting abilities. Research shows these compounds battle obesity better together than separately. One supplement gives you both. Resvinatrol Complete, made mainly from muscadine grapes, boasts 100 mg of resveratrol per serving, along with quercetin and extracts from red wine, pomegranate, and red raspberries. You can learn more about this product at the Web site *www.resvinatrolcomplete.com*.

Guard against diabetic heart problems

An antioxidant-rich supplement made from pine bark may help control diabetes and lower your blood pressure.

People who suffered from type 2 diabetes and were taking ACE inhibitors for high blood pressure were given either 125 milligrams of pycnogenol or a fake pill daily for 12 weeks. Nearly six out of 10 folks on pycnogenol were able to cut their ACE inhibitor dosage in half and still keep their blood pressure under control. Their fasting blood sugar and HbA1c levels also dropped, and their cholesterol improved. Ask your doctor if this supplement is right for you.

All-healing herb helps manage blood sugar

Traditional Chinese medicine has used ginseng for more than 2,000 years to lessen stress, relieve fatigue, improve memory, increase your strength, regulate your blood sugar, and protect your heart and blood vessels. This wildly popular Asian remedy has been revealed to the West at last, as scientific studies confirm many of its longtime uses.

For starters, both human and animal studies suggest ginseng may improve diabetes. American ginseng lowered blood sugar levels in people with this disease and helped stabilize their blood sugar after meals. Scientists say it:

- ramps up activity in the pancreas cells that make insulin.

- protects these pancreas cells from early death.

- reduces insulin resistance in muscle and fat tissue.

- guards against oxidative stress and inflammation caused by diabetes.

Korean red ginseng may battle high blood sugar, too. It improved blood sugar and insulin regulation in people with type 2 diabetes who took 2 grams of the herb three times a day before meals, in addition to their regular diabetes treatments.

Shopping for ginseng can be a bit confusing. There are two main species of this herb — American ginseng (*Panax quinquefolius L.*) and Asian ginseng (*Panax ginseng*). Asian ginseng comes in two varieties of its own. Unprocessed Asian ginseng is called "white ginseng." Asian ginseng that has been steamed and then dried is called "red ginseng."

The differences matter more than you might think, so check labels carefully. Only American and Korean Red ginseng have been shown to lower blood sugar, and American may work a little better. Regular "white" Asian ginseng, on the other hand, may actually raise your blood sugar.

Beyond that, you can buy supplements as a powdered root or extract. Read the Supplement Facts label, and make sure it meets these standards.

- For Korean Red ginseng, buy a powdered root with at least 1.5 percent total ginsenosides (15 milligrams of ginsenosides per gram of ginseng), or an extract with at least 3 percent total ginsenosides (30 milligrams per gram).

- For American ginseng, buy powdered root with at least 2 percent total ginsenosides (20 milligrams per gram), or an extract with at least 4 percent total ginsenosides (40 milligrams per gram).

Only take ginseng under your doctor's careful supervision if you have diabetes. She may need to cut back your diabetes medications. Avoid the herb entirely if you take warfarin (Coumadin) or antidepressants, since they may interact badly with ginseng.

Lastly, buyer beware. Supplement quality varies widely. An independent lab tested 18 ginseng products and found one contaminated with lead and three others that did not contain the amount of ginsenosides they claimed. To see which brands passed the quality check, visit the Web site *www.consumerlab.com*.

Heartburn meds cause dangerous deficiency

Loss of balance, muscle weakness, incontinence, moodiness, and dementia — all caused by a simple vitamin B12 deficiency that your doctor probably can't detect with a routine blood test.

Your body naturally absorbs less B12 as you age, which could leave you deficient in your golden years. Unfortunately, taking acid reflux medicines can worsen that shortage.

Proton pump inhibitors (PPIs), such as Prilosec, Prevacid, and Nexium, keep your stomach from releasing as much acid as normal. You need stomach acid to pull the B12 out of food, so using PPIs for more than two years can lead to vitamin B12 deficiency.

Luckily, you don't need stomach acid to absorb this vitamin from supplements. Some experts recommend older adults take 100 to 400 micrograms of B12 supplements daily, even if they aren't on PPIs. Ask your doctor whether you would benefit from B12 supplements.

Ease the pain of nerve damage

Neuropathy may be the most painful of all diabetes complications. And the medicines used to treat your damaged nerves don't always work and can have serious side effects. Now there's new hope from two simple supplements that may improve symptoms and even reverse some nerve damage.

Carnitine. Carnitine may help treat diabetic peripheral neuropathy (DPN) and reverse some of the nerve damage wrought by diabetes. One in 10 people with diabetes will eventually develop DPN, usually in their legs, and it gets worse with time. Tests show people suffering from diabetic complications such as DPN have lower levels of carnitine than folks with diabetes who don't have complications. Scientists suspect it helps in two ways:

- relieving pain by prompting your brain to produce more of its own natural pain relievers.

- providing extra energy to nerve cells so they can repair themselves.

In people with DPN, taking at least 2 grams (g) of L-carnitine daily eased pain, and one study found it even helped damaged nerves regrow. Your cells need carnitine to make energy, and damaged nerve cells may need more energy than usual when repairing themselves. In that sense, carnitine may literally provide the "food" those nerves need to grow.

Experts say you'll need to take at least 2 g of L-carnitine daily to ease pain and help nerve cells heal. Talk to your doctor first if you have renal failure, because you may need to start with a lower dose. It could take six months to see results, but if it helps, you can stay on it for as long as your doctor recommends.

Discuss carnitine supplements with your doctor as soon as you start to experience DPN symptoms. The earlier you begin taking it, the more likely it will help.

Alpha lipoic acid (ALA). This compound helps every cell of your body turn blood sugar into the energy that powers your body. German doctors have been prescribing it for decades for DPN.

While intravenous ALA works best for DPN, oral ALA supplements may help treat autonomic neuropathy, a condition where diabetes damages the nerves that control your internal organs, including the heart. It may also improve your blood sugar control as well as other heart, kidney, and circulatory problems caused by diabetes.

Ask your doctor how much ALA you should take every day for diabetes complications. Experts recommend anywhere from 100 to 400 mg three times a day. Don't expect to feel better right away, though. It may take several weeks to see results. In the meantime, watch your blood sugar closely. Your doctor may need to cut back your diabetes medications while you're on ALA.

Sleep supplement a heartburn hero

One pill could quiet heartburn and help you get a good night's sleep. In several small studies, people who took melatonin before bedtime got as much relief from the heartburn of gastroesophageal reflux disease (GERD) as those on proton pump inhibitors, the drugs typically used to treat GERD. What's more, melatonin may be safer for long-term use and have fewer side effects, not to mention improve your sleep quality.

You have a valve, or sphincter, at the top of your stomach that squeezes shut to keep digestive juices in your stomach from flowing up into your esophagus. In people with acid reflux, this sphincter may relax when it shouldn't, allowing stomach acid up into the esophagus. Typical heartburn remedies work by making stomach acid less acidic, so those juices don't burn. Melatonin may work a few different ways, such as:

- stopping this sphincter from relaxing at the wrong times.

- preventing the stomach from secreting corrosive digestive juice.

- protecting the esophagus from stomach-acid damage.

Taking 6 milligrams of melatonin around bedtime soothed heartburn in studies. Still, experts say you should continue your normal GERD medications for the first 40 days of melatonin treatment. After that, keep a dose of your regular medication on hand, and take it whenever symptoms reappear.

Healthful living

Melt away belly fat in 3 easy steps

Did you know that the "spare tire" you may be carrying around your waist is doing more than just slowing you down? It's also increasing your risk of heart disease, high blood pressure, type 2 diabetes, lung problems, and cancer.

Losing those extra inches around your middle will not only lower your risk for heart disease and diabetes, it will even slash your need for surgery. Women with wider waistlines are more likely to need gallbladder surgery, one of the most common operations in the United States.

Take these easy steps, and watch your belly fat melt away, your arteries clear, your blood sugar drop, and get invigorated with more energy than you ever thought possible. Start with these no-fail ways to do it safely and easily, without tough-to-follow diets.

Get moving. Walking can help flatten your stomach without gut-wrenching exercises. In a Brazilian study, people who walked 30 minutes a day, five days a week for five months shrunk their waist-lines, lowered their body mass index (BMI), shed body fat, and dropped their fasting blood sugar levels.

Start slow and set goals. Aim to walk for 10 to 30 minutes a day, three days a week, and set your own pace. Once that becomes easy, bump it up to five days a week. When you can do that, work up to walking for longer periods, first 40 then 50 minutes, until you reach an hour. Master that, and challenge yourself more by picking up the pace. By speeding up, you'll burn more calories and lose more weight while walking the same amount of time.

The point is to start with goals you can achieve and gradually build your stamina. Set impossible goals from the start, and you'll quickly lose interest. Consider investing in good, supportive walking shoes to protect your joints and back, so injuries don't derail your fitness plan.

Count your steps. Stanford researchers found that pedometer-wearers clocked about 2,000 more steps every day, or one mile more, than regular walkers. Other research shows people who use pedometers lose an extra 5 pounds a year, on average. They also cut their blood pressure enough to reduce their risk of stroke death nearly 20 percent and vascular-related death nearly 14 percent. All from wearing a device that costs as little as $10.

Set step goals to get the most benefit. For instance, put your pedometer on in the morning, and aim to walk 10,000 steps over the course of each day. Having a step goal motivated people to walk more, even when they didn't meet it.

Choose the right foods. To supercharge your weight loss, combine daily walking with an achievable diet. You'll drop pounds faster, which will boost your morale and make you more likely to stick with the program.

■ Eat smaller meals, and eat them more often. For instance, enjoy six small meals a day rather than two or three large ones.

- Aim to eat more lean protein to rev up your metabolism.

- Trim calories by eating fruits, vegetables, and whole grains in place of fatty junk foods.

Foolproof plan to a slim, trim you

Burn calories efficiently — even when resting. The secret? Just do a moderate amount of strength training exercises, then sit back and let your body do the rest.

Muscle tissue burns more calories than fat, even when you're sitting on the couch watching television. That's why weight-training exercises, push-ups, stomach crunches, and others are key to slimming down and staying that way.

- Pick a weight you can comfortably lift eight to 10 times but which still challenges your muscles. Bump up the weight once you can easily do 12 to 15 repetitions.

- Maximize your muscle by lifting the weight slowly as you breathe out, then lowering it even more slowly as you breathe in. Lowering it should take twice as long as lifting.

- Train for 20 to 30 minutes at least two days a week, preferably three.

Lighten your load to beat diabetes

More than half of people with a "normal" body weight are actually obese because they have too much fat, according to a startling Mayo Clinic study. This makes them more likely to develop metabolic syndrome, a risk factor for heart disease and type 2 diabetes.

Luckily, you can make two simple changes in your daily routine and join the ranks of the healthiest people in America. For three years, people at high risk for diabetes cut back on fat in foods and got 30 minutes of exercise five times a week. They lost enough weight to dramatically reduce their chances of diabetes. Those who melted off the most pounds slashed their risk a whopping 96 percent, but those who shed just 11 pounds still cut their risk in half.

Weight loss was key, but adding exercise to the mix aided those efforts. Even folks who lost little or no weight benefited from moving more. Exercise alone made them 44 percent less likely to get diabetes.

These changes did more to prevent this disease than medications like metformin, and the price can't be beat. Exercise can be free, not to mention fun, and you don't have to spend a lot of time doing it — even short workouts may help. Men who got on an exercise bike three times a week and "sprinted" for 30 seconds, four to six times over the course of 15 minutes, significantly improved their blood sugar control within two weeks.

Take a cue from these folks. Pick an activity you enjoy to diabetes-proof your body, even if you think you're at a healthy weight.

Gum soothes sweet cravings

Pop a stick of sugarless gum between meals if snacks keep blowing your diet. People who ate lunch, then chewed sugarless gum for a few minutes each hour for the next three hours:

- shaved 40 calories off their between-meal snack.

- generally didn't feel as hungry or crave sweet treats as much.

- had more energy in the afternoon and felt less drowsy.

3 great reasons to go for a walk

All dogs require exercise to lead balanced, healthy lives, according to Cesar Millan, world-renowned dog behavior specialist. Take a lesson from Fido. Going for a daily stroll will boost your energy, control food cravings, and reduce your risk for colon cancer.

Fights fatigue. Light workouts like walking battle fatigue better than moderate or heavy workouts. People who felt constantly tired from overworking or not sleeping enough were told to work out three times a week for six weeks.

They did either a light workout, the equivalent of taking an easy, leisurely walk; or a moderate one, akin to a fast walk on a hilly street. Both groups felt 20 percent more energetic, but the leisurely exercisers were less tired than the hard-hitting group.

Controls cravings. Going for a stroll can quell chocolate cravings, too. Taking a brisk, 15-minute walk helped chocolate lovers curb their craving and resist the treat, even when confronted with it.

Aerobic exercises like walking and jogging seem to suppress appetite, in general, by boosting your blood levels of brain-derived neurotrophic factor (BDNF). This protein helps keep nerve cells healthy, but it may also suppress appetite. One study found that exercising upped BDNF levels in overweight and obese people. The higher their BDNF, the more weight they lost and the fewer calories they ate.

Aerobic exercise also stimulates the appetite-suppressing hormone peptide YY and squashes the appetite-boosting hormone ghrelin. So go for a walk after dinner to feel satisfied and less hungry, longer.

Curbs colon cancer. Harvard researchers looked at 25 years worth of studies and concluded that people who exercise cut their chances of developing colon cancer by one-fourth.

You don't have to spend all day on a treadmill, either. "The beneficial effect of exercise holds across all sorts of activities," says the study's lead author Kathleen Wolin, a cancer prevention and control expert with the Siteman Cancer Center at Barnes-Jewish Hospital and Washington University. Jogging, bicycling, swimming, and even job-related activities like walking, lifting, and digging all seem to protect people.

Focus on fitness — not size — for longer life

How fit you are — not how fat you are — matters most if you want to live a long life. Out of more than 2,600 people over age 60, those rated as "fit" based on treadmill tests were least likely to die over the next 12 years, regardless of their weight. Those dubbed "unfit," on the other hand, were more than four times as likely to die.

You don't need to run marathons, either. Minimally fit folks were still half as likely to die as unfit people. Experts say taking a brisk walk for 30 minutes a day, most days of the week, will put almost everyone in the "fit" range.

Beauty rest beats diabetes

Don't accelerate the problems of aging. Slow them down by simply getting enough good-quality sleep. Shallow sleep, extreme insulin sensitivity, and rising diabetes risk are all typical of aging, but until now scientists didn't realize one affected the others.

People who sleep less than six hours a night are more than four times as likely to develop blood sugar problems, which can precede diabetes, as those getting six to eight hours of sleep each night. But quantity isn't the only concern. Quality matters, too.

Your brain moves through different stages of sleep during the night. The connection between sleep and blood sugar may hinge on getting plenty of deep, slow-wave sleep. Your body undergoes hormonal changes during this stage, leading researchers to suspect it's especially important for blood sugar control.

Experts used a group of healthy but sleep-deprived young people to test their theory. At night, researchers used noise to keep the young adults from slipping into deep sleep. After only three nights, the deprivation had thrown their blood sugar control out of whack.

Incredibly, their bodies reacted as if they had suddenly gained 17 to 28 pounds, and the changes were enough to qualify them as "high risk" for diabetes. Their insulin sensitivity dropped, and their glucose tolerance worsened. The less deep sleep they got, the worse their symptoms.

You don't need a scientist shaking you awake every night to end up short on this type of rest. Other factors can sabotage your sleep, too.

- Age. These tired youngsters were actually getting about the same amount of slow-wave sleep as someone 40 years older. In case you hadn't noticed, the amount of deep sleep you get each night tends to drop as you age, a change that may raise your risk for type 2 diabetes.

- Weight. Age isn't the only factor, though. Weight can worsen sleep, too. Obese people are especially prone to getting too little deep sleep, thanks in part to serious problems like sleep-disordered breathing. These troubles, in turn, could contribute to insulin resistance in obese people.

Getting more and better quality sleep, however, may help control weight in the first place, plus prevent or delay the onset of type 2 diabetes if you're at risk for it, not to mention battle high blood pressure and keep you from catching colds. Try these restful tips from the American Academy of Sleep Medicine.

■ Take care of tasks that make you worry, such as balancing the checkbook, early in the day, not last thing before bed.

■ Exercise earlier in the day, not before bedtime.

■ Stop drinking caffeine after lunch. That means caffeinated teas, too.

■ Avoid alcohol for the last six hours before bedtime.

■ Don't smoke before hitting the hay. Nicotine is a stimulant.

■ Eat large meals earlier in the evening, not later at night.

■ Only go to bed when you're sleepy. If you're not asleep after 20 minutes, get up.

■ Create relaxing bedtime rituals, like a warm bath, a special snack, reading for a few minutes, or simply brushing your teeth, to prime your mind and body for sleep.

■ Keep your bedroom dark, quiet, and slightly cool at night.

■ Sleep in bed. Don't eat, watch TV, or talk on the phone while lying there.

■ Try to get up at the same time every day to keep your body on a steady schedule.

Press secret spots to banish fatigue

Renew your vitality and replenish your energy. Just massage these secret anti-fatigue points and feel the difference right away. It may sound too good to be true, but a study from the University of Michigan shows acupressure really does revive you.

Students taking a boring, all-day class used one of two types of acupressure on themselves — they pressed either relaxation points or stimulating "alertness" points in between long bouts of sitting in a classroom. Sure enough, pressing the alertness points made them feel more awake.

It's a technique you can learn, too. Press these five places to wake up fast. Stimulate each spot, starting with the head and working your way down. For the crown, simply tap it gently for three minutes. For all the other spots, gently rub them both clockwise and counterclockwise for three minutes with your thumb or fingers.

- Put your fingers on your crown — the point in the center of the top of your head.

- Find the two bony ridges at the base of your skull. Go down 1 inch lower, then move 1.5 inches closer to the left ear on one side and the right ear on the other.

- Press into the web of each hand, in between the thumb and index finger.

- Locate the spot below each knee cap. Go four finger-widths lower, then move half an inch to the outside.

- Find the spot where your second and third toes join, then press there on the bottom of your foot, just below the ball.

Sniff a whiff to stay alert

The next time you sit down to file taxes or balance your checkbook, sniff a whiff of lavender or lemon. They'll not only make the job more pleasant, they may also keep you alert.

- You may think of lavender as a relaxing scent, but it can focus your attention, too. It's best for demanding mental tasks, where you have to concentrate for long periods of time.

- Lemon could keep you from getting tired. Students forced to do math problems had more vigor and less exhaustion over time when they smelled a lemony scent.

Simple cure for sleep apnea

It's a serious condition that may have a simple treatment, even cure. Shedding extra pounds could end sleep apnea in nearly nine out of 10 people.

People with sleep apnea stop breathing, sometimes hundreds of times, during the night. Every time they do, they wake up a little, which can leave them exhausted the next day. But the problem goes well beyond being tired. Sleep apnea can cause high blood pressure, double your risk of stroke, lead to memory loss and personality changes, and increase your chances of developing heart disease and diabetes.

You can buy dental appliances and breathing machines to help battle apnea, but the number one treatment is free — shed those extra pounds. Thirty-five sleep apnea sufferers went on a low-calorie diet and lost an average of 20 pounds in one year. Of those who lost more than 33 pounds, nine out of 10 were completely cured. Even modest weight loss can help. Six out of 10 people who lost 11 to 33 pounds were also cured.

Weight loss won't happen overnight, but you can start sleeping better now with these anti-apnea tips.

- Sleep on your side, not on your back.

- Elevate the head of your bed.

- Quit smoking.

- Avoid alcohol and sedatives before bedtime. Men, in particular, should cut back on the total amount of alcohol they drink, not just what they drink before bed.

Shiver to shed fat

Not all fat is bad. Brown fat can actually burn calories and could kick your weight loss program into high gear.

You have two types of fat in your body — white and brown. White fat stores excess energy from the foods you eat, but it also releases hormones and other compounds that can mess up your metabolism and lead to insulin resistance.

Brown fat, on the other hand, helps regulate your body temperature. It lays dormant most of the time, until you get cold. Then it leaps into action to warm you up. It's packed with mitochondria, tiny power generators inside cells. They grab fats and sugar from your bloodstream and burn them for fuel, making body heat.

Even better, it may affect your metabolism in a good way, improving your insulin sensitivity and making you less likely to gain weight with age. Having more brown fat has been linked to healthier weight, better blood sugar levels, and less overall body fat. Unfortunately, the older you get, the less brown fat you tend to have. Taking beta-blocker drugs long-term can also keep it from working, which may explain why these drugs sometimes lead to weight gain.

Being cold "turns on" its calorie-burning capabilities. In one study, people activated their brown fat by sitting in a 61-degree room for two hours, without bundling up. No one wants to get hypothermia from trying to activate their brown fat, so experts are also searching for ways to turn it on with medication. Stay tuned for break-throughs and, in the meantime, enjoy the cold weather.

6 tricks to lose weight and keep it off

You can trick yourself into feeling fuller and controlling cravings without going hungry or depriving yourself. Try these savvy strate-gies of successful dieters.

Keep a food diary. Do this and double your weight loss. People in the Weight Loss Maintenance trial who kept a food diary lost twice as much weight as those who didn't. In fact, out of 1,700 people, nearly seven in 10 dropped at least 9 pounds.

"The more food records people kept, the more weight they lost," says Jack Hollis, a researcher at Kaiser Permanente's Center for Health Research and lead author of the study. "It seems that the simple act of writing down what you eat encourages people to con-sume fewer calories."

You don't need to keep a detailed journal, however, says Keith Bachman, a doctor and member of Kaiser Permanente's Weight Management Initiative. "Keeping a food diary doesn't have to be a formal thing. Just the act of scribbling down what you eat on a Post-it note will suffice. It's the process of reflecting on what you eat that helps us become aware of our habits, and hopefully change our behavior."

Aside from keeping tabs on what went into their mouths, people in this study also:

- followed a low-fat diet based on fruits and vegetables.

- aimed for 30 or more minutes of exercise daily.

- attended weekly group support meetings.

Savor your meal. Eating slowly, taking small bites, pausing between bites, chewing your food thoroughly, and eating with a teaspoon rather than a larger soup spoon can all aid weight loss. Women who used these simple tricks ate 67 fewer calories than when they ate the same meal quickly. Plus, they felt fuller afterward. The calories add up fast. At this rate, eating slower could save an impressive 201 calories a day, if you have three meals daily.

Prepack your snacks. Breaking up large bags or boxes of snack foods into single-portion servings in resealable plastic baggies can help you eat less. Having to open a second container gives your brain the opportunity to consciously choose whether it wants to eat something or not. Otherwise, the process of snacking is mindlessly easy.

The effect wears off eventually. Your brain gets used to the packaging, so opening a second and third portion once again becomes mindless. Fight back by frequently changing the way you divvy up your snacks.

Skip the sad movie. Rent the comedy, instead. Volunteers were offered both salty popcorn and seedless grapes while watching one of two movies. Those who saw a sad film ate one-third more of the salty snack than those who watched a comedy. Researchers say people are more likely to reach for an indulgent comfort food when they're feeling blue, in order to pick themselves up.

Step on the scale. OK, so you don't really want to know how much you weigh, but checking regularly can help beat middle-age spread. People who continued to weigh in every day after they shed pounds were more likely to keep it off. Folks who avoided the scales, however, were more likely to put them back on.

Get diet help. Joining a weight-loss program that includes diet counseling can make your efforts more successful. In one study, people who continued to get counseling after they lost weight kept it off better over the next year and a half than those who skipped the counseling.

Medical alternatives

Simple new treatments for apnea sufferers

The gold standard for treating sleep apnea — the Continuous Positive Airway Pressure (CPAP) machine — can be difficult to use. As a result, many people don't stick with them. Fortunately, they aren't the only solution. Three exciting new developments may ease breathing and quiet snoring with less hassle.

Give your mouth a workout. Sixteen people with moderate sleep apnea gave their mouths a workout using tongue, soft palate, and throat exercises for 30 minutes every day. After three months, they were breathing easier, sleeping better, snoring less often and more quietly, and feeling more awake during the day, compared to sufferers who didn't do the exercises.

In obstructive sleep apnea, your upper airway collapses while you sleep, cutting off your breathing and waking you up. The researchers behind this study spent eight years developing exercises specifically to help stop this collapse. You may be able to learn them, too, by finding a speech therapist familiar with them. Ask your sleep doctor to recommend one.

Explore dental options. Oral appliances can now be used as the first line of treatment for mild to moderate sleep apnea, according to the American Academy of Sleep Medicine. But a new study suggests one mouthpiece may work for people with severe apnea, too.

Texas researchers tried the Thornton Adjustable Positioner (TAP) device in people who couldn't handle the traditional CPAP. "What we found was that many of our patients with moderate to severe sleep apnea were not adhering to standard treatment with a CPAP machine," says Paul McLornan, assistant professor in the Department of Prosthodontics at the University of Texas Dental School. Fewer than half were actually using their CPAPs, so researchers looked for another way to treat this condition.

The TAP is much smaller and fits right into your mouth. It pulls your lower jaw forward, keeping your airway open while you sleep. People in the study wore it every night, and, according to McLornan, it really worked. "We saw patients who began the study with severe sleep apnea end the study with very mild or no sleep apnea. They reported sleeping better and feeling more rested in the morning and altogether healthier." In fact, studies show people have better long-term success with oral appliances than with the standard surgery for sleep apnea, called UPPP.

The TAP isn't your only option. Other mouthpieces, such as the Dynamax, may treat mild to moderate apnea. Whichever one you choose, you'll need a dentist or orthodontist to make and fit you with it. Keep in mind, though, that oral appliances usually work best if you sleep on your back or stomach, not on your side.

Ask about implants. Pillar palatal implants mainly treat snoring, but they can also help mild to moderate sleep apnea. They're done in your doctor's office using local anesthesia. He will insert three short pieces of polyester string into the soft palate of your mouth to keep it from moving at night. Research shows it works as well as UPPP but with much less pain and a faster recovery.

The most important thing is to find something that works for you, whether it's a CPAP, dental appliance, or implant. Left untreated, obstructive sleep apnea contributes to heart attacks, coronary artery disease, high blood pressure, gastroesophageal reflux disease (GERD), and congestive heart failure. Plus, it shaves about 20 years off your life.

STOP before you have surgery

Taking a simple survey called STOP can help you avoid surgical complications and a lengthy hospital stay, and even save your life.

As many as one in four people suffer from sleep apnea, but nine out of 10 don't know it. Those are dangerous odds, especially when you undergo surgery. People with obstructive sleep apnea are more likely to suffer intubation problems, postoperative complications, and death following surgery. They also tend to have longer hospital stays and higher rates of admission to Intensive Care.

However, if the anesthesiologist knows or suspects you have sleep apnea, he can choose techniques and equipment better suited to your situation, as well as make certain the surgery happens in a hospital equipped to deal with potential complications.

Most hospitals and clinics don't screen people for sleep apnea before surgery, largely because there hasn't been an easy way to do so — until now. Experts have developed four yes/no questions, called the STOP survey, that can help your doctors and anesthesiologist determine if you have sleep apnea. Test yourself by answering these STOP questions.

■ Do you snore loudly (louder than talking or loud enough to be heard through closed doors)?

- Do you often feel tired, fatigued, or sleepy during the daytime?

- Has anyone observed you stop breathing during your sleep?

- Do you have or are you being treated for high blood pressure?

If you answered "yes" to two or more questions, there is a good chance you suffer from sleep apnea. That chance goes up even further if you:

- are male.

- are over age 50.

- have a body mass index (BMI) above 35.

- have a thick neck more than 40 centimeters (15.75 inches) around.

Let your doctor know if you think you have sleep apnea, even if you aren't planning any surgeries. By treating the condition, you'll live a longer, healthier life.

Nondrug solution to nausea

Wearing a wristband can quell post-surgery nausea. So says a review of 40 studies on acupressure and acupuncture. Pressing the P6 point, 2 inches up your arm from your inner wrist, seems to be the key. It's the same spot targeted by wristbands sold for motion sickness. In one study, stimulating this point worked about as well as drugs in relieving nausea and vomiting, plus reduced the need for rescue doses of anti-nausea medicine.

Easier screenings for colon cancer

No one enjoys getting colonoscopies, but new tests and techniques may soon make them rarer and more tolerable.

Take a simpler test. Too many people put off their colonoscopy because it is unpleasant. And although it's the preferred way to screen for colon cancer, a test is only as good as people's willingness to get it. Unfortunately, the more popular, noninvasive FOBT (fecal occult blood test) is simply not very good at catching colon cancer early. That's a problem, because early detection boosts your chances of survival.

Thankfully, scientists may have discovered an easier way to check for this deadly disease. Most people with colon cancer have high levels of the protein CD24 in their blood. Now, new research shows that a simple blood test can check your CD24 levels and reliably catch cancer in its early stages.

Get better biopsies. Your doctor may still want you to have a colonscopy, especially if the CD24 test is positive. That's where a new device known as a confocal endomicroscopy system (CFM) comes in. It's a high-powered probe that can not only spot colon polyps but also tell if they're benign or cancerous — before removing them for biopsy. As a result, you'll have fewer needless polyp removals and biopsies.

Book it in the morning. Schedule your screening first thing in the morning, while the doctor is still fresh and alert. Doctors were more likely to catch and remove precancerous polyps during morning colonscopies, compared to afternoon ones, according to one study. The likelihood of spotting dangerous polyps dropped for every hour later people were scheduled.

Stay on schedule. The type of screening you get, whether a colonoscopy, flexible sigmoidoscopy, CT colonography, or fecal test, matters less than whether you stick with the recommended screening schedule. You may not need routine screening once you turn 76. The U.S. Preventive Services Task Force says that, for most people, the risks of colon cancer tests start to outweigh the benefits after age 75.

Different types of screening methods have different schedules. Discuss your risk factors, medical history, and test options with your doctor to find the right one for you.

Chew gum to speed recovery

Enjoying a few sticks of gum can help you bounce back faster from colorectal surgery. New research shows that gum chewers recovered about one day sooner than people who didn't chew gum. It may not necessarily shorten your hospital stay, but it may help your bowels and digestive tract get back to normal faster.

6 reasons to consider weight-loss surgery

It's controversial, but it could save lives. Bariatric, or weight-loss, surgery can help people who haven't lost weight the old-fashioned way, not to mention quickly stem diabetes, heart problems, and other obesity-related conditions.

- Weight-loss surgery cured type 2 diabetes in three out of four people in one study and slashed the risk of diabetes-related death a whopping 92 percent in another.

- Obese people who had bariatric surgery were half as likely to die from coronary artery disease and 43 percent less likely to suffer a heart attack as those who didn't.

- The procedure cured high blood pressure in six out of 10 obese people and improved cholesterol levels in seven out of 10.

- Eighty-five percent of obese sleep-apnea sufferers were cured after bariatric surgery.

- Obese people who underwent gastric bypass surgery were 60 percent less likely to die from cancer.

- Getting gastric bypass surgery made obese people 40 percent less likely to die over the next seven years, in one study, and 89 percent less likely in another.

Not everyone is a good candidate for surgery, but people who are morbidly obese and have both diabetes and metabolic syndrome may benefit most. Medicare will even cover these three bariatric procedures if you have a body mass index (BMI) of 35 or higher and have:

- at least one obesity-related health condition, such as type 2 diabetes.

- not been able to lose weight with other weight-loss treatments.

Laparoscopic adjustable gastric banding (LAGB). This procedure shrinks your stomach to a small pouch roughly the size of a thumb, forcing you to eat less. The pouch size can be increased or decreased, depending on how fast you're losing weight.

Roux-en-Y gastric bypass (RYGBP). It not only shrinks your stomach to a small pouch but also reroutes your digestive tract so the stomach empties directly into the middle portion of the small intestine. You'll feel full after small meals, plus absorb fewer calories from food.

Biliopancreatic Diversion with Duodenal Switch (BPD/DS). A combination procedure much like RYGBP, it creates a larger stomach pouch, allowing you to eat more normal-sized meals. The pouch hooks up to your intestines farther down, closer to the colon, limiting the calories and nutrients you absorb even more.

Age can increase the chances of surgical complications, but research shows that risk drops substantially if you have an experienced surgeon perform the procedure. Hospitals play a role, too. The more procedures one does, the fewer complications and deaths. Look for Bariatric Surgery Centers of Excellence, or Level 1 Bariatric Surgery Centers, for experienced doctors and hospitals.

Even if everything goes smoothly, you will most likely suffer some side effects and risks from any type of weight-loss surgery.

- Vomiting, nausea, heartburn, gastritis, and trouble swallowing are common complications.

- Rapid weight loss following surgery can boost your risk for gallstones.

- You may need to take prescribed vitamins and minerals for life to avoid malnutrition.

- As many as one in four people will need repeat or corrective surgery after the first procedure.

- You will have to chew your food thoroughly and eat smaller meals.

- Your new stomach may not be able to handle food and liquids at the same time.

- You won't be able to eat as much fat or sugar, or drink as much alcohol, as before. Avoid deep-fried foods, fast food, and other high-fat, high-sugar treats.

Procedures which reroute your digestive tract, such as RYGBP and BPD/DS, tend to result in more weight loss, but they carry bigger risks for nutritional deficiencies in the long run.

For some people, surgery alone isn't enough. About 10 percent don't lose enough weight, or regain much of it, especially if they continue snacking on high-calorie foods and don't exercise. You'll have to change your lifestyle, not just go under the knife, to make weight loss stick.

Hormone therapy made safer

Gallbladder disease becomes more common after menopause, and hormone therapy doesn't help. The higher your hormone dose, the higher your risk of gallbladder disease. But a major new study found that getting hormones through a skin patch or gel put women less at risk than taking it as a pill. Ask your doctor which therapy is right for you.

New drugs rev up weight loss

Surgery isn't the only option if you're struggling to lose weight. The new drug tesofensine may help you drop twice as many pounds as current weight-loss medications, by both suppressing hunger and making you feel fuller and more satisfied. It's still being tested and is not yet available, but other medicines are. Current drugs come in three types:

Appetite suppressants. These make you feel less hungry and more full by boosting brain chemicals involved in mood and appetite. One drug, sibutramine, can be taken for up to one year, while others, including phentermine, phendimetrazine, and diethylpropion, can only be taken for three months at a time.

Your doctor won't prescribe appetite suppressants if you have heart disease, high blood pressure, an irregular heartbeat, an overactive thyroid, glaucoma, or a history of stroke.

Fat blockers. Also known as lipase inhibitors, fat blockers stop the enzyme lipase from breaking down fat in food. Your body can't absorb the fat, so it gets eliminated with other waste, sparing you those calories. The fat-blocker orlistat (Alli), comes in both prescription and over-the-counter strengths, although new research does link it to liver damage. Follow these tips to make the most of this medicine.

- Don't rely on orlistat alone to melt off the pounds. You're supposed to exercise and cut back calories while on it.

- Trim the fat from your diet, since it can worsen the drug's side effects.

- Take a multivitamin at least two hours before taking orlistat. The medicine blocks your body from absorbing some nutrients in food.

Off-label drugs. Some antidepressants also suppress your appetite and may help you lose weight for up to six months. However, people usually start regaining the weight after that, even if they stay on the medicine. One antidepressant, buproprion, may keep the weight off for up to a year.

Pills are no magic bullet for getting or staying slim. Weight-loss drugs only help you drop an average of 10 pounds more than you would lose on your own through healthy eating and exercise. And some medications stop working as your body adapts to them.

That said, even short-term weight loss can slash your risk of other diseases. Studies show prescription weight-loss medicines may help improve blood pressure, cholesterol, triglycerides, and your body's ability to use blood sugar. The bottom line — talk to your doctor about medicine if you simply can't shed enough weight with lifestyle changes.

Everyday pill helps curb disease

You could can colon cancer and beat diabetes with just a few cents a day, thanks to the humble aspirin and its relatives.

Fight back against cancer. Scientists have known for years that people who take aspirin are less likely to get colon cancer, but new research shows this everyday drug may help treat it, too.

Most, but not all, colon tumors churn out too much of the inflammatory enzyme COX-2. Aspirin has the power to stop cells from producing COX-2. In the latest study, people who began taking the pain reliever after being diagnosed with stage I, II, or III colon cancer cut their risk of dying in half. People whose tumors produced COX-2 benefited most, with a 61 percent drop in their chances of dying.

Experts warn the study was observational and doesn't actually prove anything. They want to see more research before recommending aspirin and other COX-2 inhibitors for colon cancer treatment. For now, side effects such as gastrointestinal irritation and bleeding make it too risky, but with advancements, this inexpensive little pill may one day become standard treatment for some types of colon cancer.

Discuss aspirin therapy with your doctor first if you have colon cancer or a high risk for it. Look at the pros and cons together as well as proper dosage.

Get a grip on diabetes. An aspirin-like drug helped lower blood sugar levels in obese people who were otherwise healthy. Researchers suspect salicylates like aspirin make the beta-cells in your pancreas produce more insulin.

A separate study found that low doses of aspirin combated diabetes especially well when taken alongside the diabetes drug rosiglitazone. Aspirin could also help combat the higher heart disease risk you face if you have diabetes.

Private talk: living without limits 5

Ditch cancer with 5 fabulous foods

You don't have to eat exotic fruits and vegetables to stay cancer-free. The natural plant chemicals in these five delicious, everyday foods will give you a fighting chance to head off breast cancer.

Make apples a daily treat. Apples keep the doctor away with more than a dozen protective compounds called triterpenoids. Lab studies show these phytochemicals keep cancer cells from growing. Since they're found mostly in an apple's peel, eat the fruit whole or drink cloudy apple juice or cider. Make apples one of the five to 12 servings of fruits and vegetables you eat every day.

Enjoy the many benefits of grapes. This fruit has a natural antioxidant in its skin called resveratrol. It helps block the growth of breast tumors by preventing estrogen from starting the process that leads to cancer. You'll find resveratrol in red wine, blueberries, cranberries, and peanuts, but the real powerhouse is red and purple grape juice.

Besides slowing the growth of tumors, this tasty beverage can reduce blood pressure and cholesterol, plus it may even boost your brainpower. Resveratrol's benefits come from its powerful antioxidant effects.

Relish the crunch of cauliflower. Researchers found that women in China who ate more cruciferous vegetables, such as turnips and Chinese cabbage, had less chance of developing breast cancer than other women. What's so great about these veggies? They're full of isothiocyanates like sulforaphane. These phytochemicals work like cancer drugs to stop tumor cells from dividing and growing. Women in the study who also had a particular gene variation enjoyed even greater protection. Good sources of isothiocyanates include cauliflower, broccoli, and cabbage.

Open up the olive oil. Its healthy fats help your heart, but this liquid gold also sports a treasure trove of cancer-fighting polyphenols. These phytochemicals were found to effectively block the breast cancer gene HER2 in a lab study. You'll get the most polyphenols from extra virgin olive oil, which is less refined than other types. Another great source is green tea. Add a splash of lemon juice, and your body will absorb even more cancer-fighters from the tea.

Treat yourself to walnuts. Phytosterols, literally "plant sterols," are fatty compounds in some nuts, including walnuts and pistachios. Research in mice found that eating more walnuts may cut your risk of developing breast cancer. Walnuts also provide lots of omega-3 fatty acids and antioxidants, which battle this disease, too. Skip the cookies, and snack on these tasty treats.

Egg-cellent way to crack breast cancer risk

The incredible, edible egg has lots of protein, and it tastes great. Now it has another great thing going for it — choline.

Choline — pronounced ko-lean — is a nutrient your body needs to help cells function, including brain and nerve cells. Research has found it may help your memory and protect your heart as well as lower your risk for breast cancer. In one study, women who ate six or more eggs a week were 44 percent less likely to develop breast cancer compared to those who ate two or less.

Before menopause, the natural estrogens in women's bodies help make choline from scratch. But postmenopausal women, along with men, need to get their choline from food.

One egg yolk has about 125 milligrams (mg), more than a quarter of a woman's daily requirement. If you eat two scrambled eggs for breakfast, you're halfway to getting your choline for the day. Add a cup of coffee for an extra choline boost. Make an effort to include cauliflower, wheat germ, liver, and pistachios in your diet, and you'll get more than enough of this important nutrient.

Why you should skip the burger and fries

You can cut your risk of breast cancer simply by keeping these two items off your menu. Here's why.

French fries are a major source of trans fats, and research shows they raise your risk of breast cancer. Trans fats occur naturally in red meats and dairy products and synthetically in hydrogenated oils — the kind many restaurants use to cook their fries. If your restaurant meal comes with a side item, pick a fresh fruit cup or salad instead.

The problem with red meat may be its saturated fat. Experts say eating more of this type of fat raises the estrogen in your system, which also ups your risk for breast cancer. Multiple studies show women who eat more red meat and fat are more likely to develop this disease. Try eating chicken or fish instead of a burger.

Get the scoop on soy

Several Asian studies have found that women who eat the most soy, especially when they're young, have the lowest risk of breast cancer. Experts say soy's protection comes from its phytoestrogens — plant estrogens — including isoflavones. Other research supports the theory that women who eat more soy foods have a lower risk of breast cancer. A University of Southern California analysis of eight studies concluded that soy, in the amounts eaten in Asian countries, may have a protective effect.

But the research on soy is not all good. Some animal studies show the opposite — that isoflavones fuel the growth of cancer cells that feed off estrogen. Other studies warn that soy may harm your memory as you age. See the story "Smarter ways to enjoy soy" on page 15 in *Age-proof your brain* for the latest findings on how soy foods affect your memory.

Your best bet is to ask your doctor before you add soy to your diet to see if it's a good choice for you. If she approves, you can try soy-based meat and dairy substitutes, like soy milk and cheese; tofu; and foods like miso soup and edamame. Moderation is best. One study suggested that eating 10 milligrams of isoflavones every day — a typical serving of tofu — may be beneficial for breast cancer protection.

'Miracle' fats keep your prostate young

One in six men in the United States will get prostate cancer. Be one of those five healthy guys by adding powerful prostate protection to your diet. Unfortunately, most men never think much about the prostate, a gland that surrounds the urethra, the tube that takes urine out of the body. But prostate cancer is the most common, nonskin cancer among men in the United States.

New research shows eating foods rich in omega-3 fatty acids may prevent prostate cancer. You can get these amazing fats from eating fatty fish or flaxseeds. One study found that men who ate more omega-3 fatty acids — especially those who ate dark fish, like salmon, at least once a week — had less risk of developing aggressive prostate cancer. The protective effect of the fats was even stronger among men who had the COX-2 gene type that puts them at higher risk for prostate cancer. This fact made researchers think the fats work on the enzymes that affect COX-2, a known inflammatory gene.

Another study found that supplementing the diet with ground flaxseed daily also slows the growth of prostate tumors. What's more, sticking to a low-fat diet gives you extra protection. There is some concern that flaxseed oil — but not flaxseeds — may actually encourage prostate tumors to grow. If you've already been diagnosed with prostate cancer, check with your doctor before making any changes to your diet.

Surprisingly, you can send your risk of prostate cancer to the cellar if you lower your cholesterol levels while you raise the amount of omega-3s in your diet. Taking a cholesterol-lowering drug, like eze-timibe (Zetia), seems to stop the growth of blood vessels that feed tumors. But if you eat more fish and flaxseed with omega-3s, you'll also keep cholesterol from building up in your arteries. That lets you kill two birds with one stone, just by increasing these fats in your diet.

Other research has found that men who have had prostate cancer and eat a diet high in saturated fats — like the kind in beef, butter, cheese, and ice cream — have a higher risk of having their cancer return. That gives you one more reason to choose fish over a hamburger.

Eating fish rich in omega-3 fatty acids is good for more than your prostate. Just two servings a week fight depression, heart attack, stroke, diabetes, and colon cancer. These good fats are known to cut excess inflammation in your body, which affects how your brain works and changes your risk factors for chronic conditions like heart disease and cancer, along with diabetes and its side effects. Keep your prostate — and the rest of your body — young with extra servings of these miracle fats.

Simple help for a leaky bladder

Watch what you eat and drink, and you may stop urine leakage caused by irritation of your bladder lining. This may help solve the problem of urinary incontinence. Avoid these foods to cut down on irritation.

- chocolate

- tomatoes

- citrus juice and fruits

- spicy foods

- alcoholic beverages

- soft drinks with caffeine

- milk and milk products

- sugar, corn syrup, honey, and artificial sweeteners

- coffee, even decaf

- tea

But don't limit the amount of water you drink. Although drinking less means your body makes less urine, it also means urine is more concentrated, which can also irritate the bladder lining. That creates a vicious cycle.

3 super fruits for men's health

Two major age-related concerns of the "tougher" sex are prostate cancer and erectile dysfunction (ED). Natural chemicals in certain fruits may help with both problems.

Pomegranate. This feisty holiday favorite boasts ellagitannins — polyphenols that work as antioxidants. These natural chemicals are digested into urolithins, which fight prostate cancer. Men with prostate cancer who drank 8 ounces of pomegranate juice daily saw a slower rise in their PSA scores, the marker that shows the presence of cancer.

Men in their 60s and 70s may be able to drink pomegranate juice and slow the growth of prostate tumors to the point where they can avoid cancer treatment. In one study, the average time it took PSA scores to double went from about 15 months to five years for the men drinking pomegranate juice daily. But this benefit has only been shown with prostate cancer that has not spread.

Antioxidants in pomegranate juice also helped men with mild to moderate ED enjoy improved function. Just 8 ounces a day for four weeks helped. The antioxidants mop up free radicals in your body that can disrupt circulation, including blood flow to your private parts. This effect on circulation is also why pomegranate juice is thought to be good for your heart.

Many studies have used POM Wonderful brand of juice, and this company also funded some of the research. But POM Wonderful isn't cheap — you'll probably pay around $3 for each 8 ounce glass. Check your grocery store for cheaper brands, such as R.W. Knudsen or Lakewood.

Watermelon. The deep redness of watermelons, just like tomatoes, comes from lycopene, an antioxidant that protects both the prostate and heart. Lycopene's cancer-busting action comes from its ability to block the action of dangerous free radicals, which can damage your cells.

But if ED is your concern, you'll be glad watermelons have citrulline, an amino acid that works like Viagra to relax blood vessels and improve sexual function in men. Dr. Bhimu Patil of the Texas A&M Fruit and Vegetable Improvement Center explains watermelon's beneficial effects on ED. "Watermelon may not be as organ specific as Viagra," Patil says, "but it's a great way to relax blood vessels without any drug side effects."

Cranberry. These tart treats contain several phytochemicals — natural plant chemicals — believed to prevent cancer of the prostate, breast, colon, and lungs. First, there are anthocyanins, dark-colored pigments that give cranberries their crimson hue. These antioxidants repair and protect the DNA in your cells to block tumor growth. Other phytochemicals, including quercetin, proanthocyanidins, and ursolic acid, work together to thwart cancer.

Secret to a healthy prostate

Next time someone offers you a second helping of veggies, take it. Your prostate will thank you. Many men wage war against an enlarged prostate, called benign prostatic hyperplasia (BPH), as they age. But eating your veggies may keep the problem at bay. Researchers found that middle-age men and older who ate the most vegetables had fewer symptoms of BPH.

Men fared best on diets high in certain antioxidants — beta carotene, lutein, and vitamin C. Allium vegetables, like onions and garlic, were also found to be powerful protectors. Antioxidants from the vegetables are thought to limit the oxidative damage of BPH, which is caused by unstable molecules called free radicals.

Improve your odds with natural cancer fighters

An anti-cancer warrior is waiting for you in the produce aisle. This powerful plant compound, known as sulforaphane, may help fight off cancers of the bladder and prostate. You can get this and similar compounds in cruciferous vegetables, like broccoli. If you're not a fan of broccoli, how about cauliflower, cabbage, brussels sprouts, kale, turnips, collard greens, or radishes?

All these cruciferous veggies have lots of isothiocyanates — phyto-chemicals that lower your risk of bladder cancer. Sulforaphane, a type of isothiocyanate, boosts your immune system's ability to fight off disease. These natural antioxidants help enzymes bring on apoptosis — planned death — of cancer cells. Researchers found that eating lots of cruciferous vegetables was linked to a 29 percent lower risk of bladder cancer.

Other researchers compared the cancer-fighting ability of broccoli with peas, focusing on prostate cancer. Men at risk of prostate cancer ate either broccoli or peas — about two large servings every week for a year. At the end of the study, fewer of the broccoli-eating guys had signs of prostate cancer. Experts say it's the isothio-cyanates at work.

But pay attention to food preparation. The best way to get the most of these helpful natural chemicals is to eat your broccoli raw. Cooking it lowers the amount of isothiocyanates available to your body. A small study in the Netherlands found that men who ate broccoli raw rather than cooked absorbed more of the sulforaphane. And the heads of broccoli contain more sulforaphane than the stems, so it's best to eat all of the broccoli rather than broccoli slaw, made from the stems. In the end, however, even broccoli stems have more of this compound than other vegetables.

Kidney stone myth busters

Forget everything you thought you knew about eating to prevent kidney stones. New research shows you may not have to give up the foods you love after all.

Myth: Meat is a no-no. Some experts say to limit the amount of protein you get from meat, but the research isn't crystal clear. A review of studies found evidence on both sides, but no strong case against eating meat. Still, fish may be your best bet. Research shows people who've had problems with calcium stones can avoid them by taking supplements of eicosapentaenoic acid (EPA), one of the omega-3 fatty acids in fish oil.

Myth: Salt is a villain. Evidence is weak on this one, and it may depend on the individual. One study found that people who cut back on protein and salt but ate a typical amount of calcium had less oxalate in their urine. That's a sign of lower risk for kidney stones. Other research found that adding more salt to the diet — in the form of sodium supplements — encouraged people to drink more water. Ask your doctor for advice on whether salt will hurt or help you.

Myth: Dairy products are dangerous. Not so. Lots of calcium from food or supplements doesn't seem to raise your risk. In fact, some research shows calcium from dairy foods may help protect you from stones.

Myth: Coffee and tea are off limits. You can widen your range of beverages to include these favorites. It's a myth that the caffeine in coffee dehydrates your system, and researchers found coffee may actually be protective. The problem with black tea is its oxalate content, but that may only affect people who tend to form calcium oxalate stones.

But do follow the tried-and-true advice to drink lots of water to dilute your urine. Drink enough to produce two quarts of water every 24 hours. Lemonade is also a good choice.

Surprising cause of kidney damage

Here's another reason to choose water over sugary soda pop. You'll save your kidneys.

Women who drink two or more sugary sodas per day have a higher risk of developing kidney damage, measured by testing for albuminuria, or protein in the urine. Drinking one soda a day or drinking diet soda doesn't increase risk. Researchers suspect it's the high fructose corn syrup in sodas that does the damage.

Other natural remedies

Supplement warning no woman should ignore

Check the supplements in your cabinet if you're about to undergo treatment for breast cancer. Some 40 percent of people who have cancer take vitamins or other supplements, but these may interfere with the drugs that treat your cancer. Problem is, as many as two-thirds of those who use unproven therapies don't tell their doctors. Here are three that could cause problems.

Vitamin E. Because it's an antioxidant, vitamin E may protect tumor cells as well as healthy cells from the types of treatment that would kill the cancer. Research shows you shouldn't take antioxidant supplements while you're getting any kind of chemotherapy or radiation treatment. Experts used to think vitamin E might help protect against the side effects of chemotherapy, but studies have not borne this out. And vitamin E supplements seem to interfere with tamoxifen, a drug commonly used to block estrogen in hormone-positive breast cancer tumors.

Vitamin C. Vitamin C is also an antioxidant, so it, too, may protect cancer cells. One study found that vitamin C seems to shield a cancer cell's mitochondria, or power plant, so chemotherapy can't kill it.

Genistein. This supplement is a soy isoflavone and a phytoestrogen, or plant estrogen, that works like that hormone in your body. Many women take genistein to control hot flashes and other symptoms of menopause. But genistein interferes with a class of anti-cancer drugs called aromatase inhibitors, including one called Letrozole. Some postmenopausal women fighting cancer take these drugs to lower their levels of estrogen.

The bottom line is, don't take supplements during cancer treatment without consulting your doctor.

Ditch the itch with probiotics

An over-the-counter probiotic pill may help prevent your next yeast infection.

Probiotics are friendly bacteria that can help your body in many ways. One of them is to keep unwanted yeast and bacteria from overcolonizing your personal spaces. The supplement Fem-Dophilus contains two strains of *Lactobacillus* bacteria known to treat vaginal infections. It works by coating your vaginal lining to keep unwanted bacteria from growing there, along with repopulating the vagina with good microflora.

One capsule daily will help you avoid vaginal infections, but if you suffer from them only occasionally, you can take as needed. Using Fem-Dophilus during and after a course of antibiotic treatment may be especially helpful because the probiotics restore the good microflora as the drug kills off the bad.

Outsmart kidney stones

Know your stones — kidney stones, that is. Phosphorus supplements may help keep you from another painful attack, but you need to know what kind of stones your body forms. Otherwise, the supplements may actually cause more problems.

The mineral phosphorus occurs naturally in foods like milk, cheese, peanut butter, and dried beans. You'll sometimes see phosphorus referred to by its common form, phosphate. Taking sodium phosphate or potassium phosphate, two types of salts made from this mineral, may prevent kidney stones if you have too much calcium in your urine, a condition called hypercalciuria. It's also helpful if you tend to form kidney stones made of calcium oxalate.

A urinary tract infection may spur the formation of magnesium-ammonium phosphate, or struvite, stones. If your stones contain phosphates, then taking phosphorus supplements will simply add fuel to the fire and cause your body to form more stones. Try to save your kidney stone after it passes so the doctor can analyze it to see what type it is.

If he gives the OK for phosphorus supplements, look for "sodium phosphate" or "potassium phosphate" on the label. Common brands include K-Phos and Neutra-Phos. You'll typically take the supplement four times a day, preferably after you eat. Ask your doctor for specific advice.

Hidden danger of multivitamins

Just when it seems you can rely on a vitamin or mineral to help ward off a scary part of aging, researchers find it's not so simple. Experts speculated that the mineral selenium and vitamin E might help prevent prostate cancer. Unfortunately, the Selenium and Vitamin E Cancer Prevention Trial (SELECT), a huge study of more than 35,000 men, found that's probably not true.

The study was supposed to continue for seven years, but it was stopped early when researchers noticed the supplements brought no benefit — and they may even cause harm. Slightly more of the men taking vitamin E were getting prostate cancer, and slightly more of those taking selenium were developing diabetes. Men in the study took 200 micrograms of selenium and 400 international units (IUs) of vitamin E, alone or together. That's several times the amount found in a typical multivitamin.

Other research has brought up questions about multivitamins, those all-purpose pills most people think are perfectly harmless. One study found that regular use of multivitamins won't affect whether you'll get prostate cancer, but men classified as "heavy users" have a higher risk of the disease. Heavy users took multivitamins more than seven times a week. The danger was greatest for heavy users with a family history of prostate cancer, as well as for heavy users who took additional selenium, beta carotene, and zinc supplements.

Many health professionals say there's a better way to stay healthy. Aim for a balanced diet — with fruits, vegetables, whole grains, healthy fats, lean meat, and low-fat dairy — to get all the nutrients you need, and don't rely on a pill to prevent cancer.

OTC aids for impotence

Impotence, also known as erectile dysfunction (ED), becomes more common as men get older. One survey found that 44 percent of men over age 50 had experienced this frustrating condition. If it's a recurring problem for you, ask your doctor about taking a prescription drug. Although many men prefer taking supplements, there's not a lot of research on most of these so-called remedies, but you may find one that helps you feel virile again.

Remember, herbs and other supplements are not regulated by the U.S. Food and Drug Administration (FDA), so there's no guarantee they contain the ingredients they claim. Some supplements may interact with your prescription drugs, so be sure to ask your doctor before you try them.

- **B vitamins.** Along with helping your ED, B vitamins may lower your blood level of homocysteine. High levels of this amino acid sometimes signal heart disease. The connection makes sense, since ED is often related to heart disease.

- **Yohimbine.** Made from the bark of an African tree, this herbal remedy improves blood flow and does its job for up to 75 percent of men who try it. Usual dose is 5 to 10 milligrams (mg).

- Ginseng. Both American ginseng and the Korean red variety are herbs used to treat impotence. Experts think the active ingredients are ginsenosides, which may both affect the central nervous system and help tissues in the penis to expand.

- Pycnogenol. This extract from the bark of a French pine tree is also thought to treat asthma, heart disease, and diabetes. If you want to try pycnogenol for ED, some experts recommend taking 120 mg daily.

- L-arginine. Your body uses this amino acid to produce nitric oxide, important for the muscles that help blood vessels function.

- Ginkgo. Some herbal experts believe this Asian herb improves sexual function, but it may cause bleeding and convulsions if you take too much.

Healthful living

Calm your overactive bladder

Police in Mobile, Ala., arrested an 81-year-old woman after she resorted to squatting behind bushes in a local park when she couldn't make it to the restroom. She said she had an incontinence problem — no laughing matter for many older women.

Urinary incontinence, or a problem controlling your bladder, is common among women middle age and older. You're more likely to have problems if you've been pregnant, have diabetes, are overweight, or have other health problems. Men with prostate problems may also suffer from incontinence. Surgery or other medical procedures may ease incontinence. But even the best surgeries come with the risk of complications, including infections and new urinary symptoms.

Before you rush to have surgery, see what you can do to solve the problem on your own.

Do Kegel exercises. These exercises strengthen the muscles of the pelvic floor, which can be weakened or damaged by childbirth or aging. Kegels are especially helpful with stress incontinence. Try squeezing the muscles you use to stop urinating. Hold them tight for about 10 seconds, and then relax for the same amount of time. Do this 10 times. Aim for three sets of exercises daily.

Lose weight if you need to. Gaining weight around your midsection means there's added pressure on your bladder and pelvic area, increasing your risk for incontinence. Overweight women who lost just 8 percent of their body weight found they had half the episodes of incontinence. That's a big improvement for a fairly small weight loss.

Watch your fluid intake. Volume in equals volume out. Researchers found that people with overactive bladder problems could reduce their symptoms by lowering the amount they drank by 25 percent. Not surprisingly, when others increased the amount they drank, they had more problems. Be sure to drink enough to avoid dehydration.

Explore the mind-body connection. Ask your doctor about professional help for the mental component of the problem. This could mean biofeedback training, which can help with urge incontinence, or cognitive therapy, using guided imagery or deep-breathing exercises to calm an overactive bladder.

4 smart ways to beat bladder cancer

You worry about lung cancer, skin cancer, and prostate cancer. But tumors can also grow in your bladder, especially in men. Follow these good-health tips to avoid this costly disease.

Drink lots of water. Research shows people who drink water — as little as five or six glasses a day — have a lower risk of bladder and colon cancer. Other studies find drinking more fluids of all kinds lowers your risk. Experts believe that putting more fluids through your urinary tract helps flush out cancer-causing substances.

Heed the call of nature. You can also lower your risk by urinating when you feel the urge — even if it means you have to get up at night. Again, getting those cancer-causing toxins out of your system quickly means they don't stay in contact with your bladder.

Don't smoke. This bad habit is to blame for up to half of all bladder cancers. If you quit smoking, your risk goes down by 40 percent within four years.

Avoid chlorine. The byproducts of chlorine in water, trihalomethanes (THM), can leach through your skin and may increase your risk of bladder cancer. Try to limit your exposure to chlorinated water through drinking it or swimming or bathing in it.

Choose gentle approach for cancer care

Go-getter tactics, like eating a low-calorie diet and getting vigorous exercise, are recommended to help prevent breast cancer. But if you've been diagnosed and are undergoing treatment, a gentler approach may be better. Progressive muscle relaxation, massage, and tai chi are all ways to reduce tension and boost your immune response. That may help your body fight off the cancer so you can heal and get back to your life.

Treat BPH without risky drugs

Simple changes in your daily routine may help ease the symptoms of benign prostatic hyperplasia (BPH), an enlarged prostate. That's the gland in men that surrounds the urethra, or the tube that takes urine out of your body. BPH is common among men as they age, and it can interfere with urination. You may notice a weak or sputtering stream when you urinate due to the gland pressing against the urethra or causing muscle spasms. BPH may also cause you to get up to urinate at night — maybe even several times.

Here are some tricks to deal with these symptoms and make your life more comfortable.

- Lose weight if you need to. Research shows that men who carry extra weight are more likely to have BPH symptoms. Add in diabetes or trouble controlling your blood sugar levels, and your risk is even greater.

- Stay active. Getting more physical activity, either at work or at play, can reduce BPH symptoms. Experts say physical activity affects several hormones, which control BPH and prostate growth.

- Don't delay urinating when you need to go, and limit the amount you drink after 7 p.m.

- Limit your use of over-the-counter antihistamines and decon-gestants, which can keep the muscles around your bladder from relaxing.

- Practice Kegel exercises to strengthen the muscles of your pelvic floor.

- Stay warm. Cold weather can affect your sympathetic nervous system and bring on symptoms.

- Watch your numbers. Keep your cholesterol, blood pressure, and blood sugar at healthy levels.

Prostate cancer news you can use

Overweight men have a higher risk of prostate cancer than their lean buddies. And that's not all — tests and treatments seem to work better for the slender.

- Researchers found that overweight men who lost more than 11 pounds lowered their risk of developing an aggressive form of prostate cancer.

- Men diagnosed with prostate cancer who are overweight or obese have a higher risk of dying of the disease than those at a healthy weight. Your risk is even higher if you're both overweight and have a high blood level of C-peptide, a marker of insulin secretion.

- Being overweight also means radiation therapy for your prostate cancer may be less effective.

- Obesity lowers your PSA readings. If you're overweight and have a slightly elevated PSA level, you may be at greater risk than a thin man with the same number.

Little-known cause of kidney stones

You have a higher chance for kidney stones if you have metabolic syndrome. That's a fancy term for the combination of obesity, diabetes, and high blood pressure. Experts think it's because people with metabolic syndrome tend to create urine that's more acidic. It also may be due to eating too much protein and sodium. Get your weight and blood pressure under control, and you may avoid the pain of kidney stones.

Medical alternatives

One a day cuts breast cancer

The daily aspirin you take for your heart may also ward off breast cancer.

Researchers found that middle-age women who took a daily aspirin were 16 percent less likely to develop the estrogen receptor-positive type of breast cancer. Experts aren't sure how aspirin protects, and they noticed it didn't affect risk for other types of breast cancer. Another study found women who regularly take either aspirin or ibuprofen (Advil) had a lower risk of breast cancer.

But the experts at the American Cancer Society don't recommend you start taking daily aspirin merely to prevent breast cancer. Aspirin carries risks, like bleeding, and it's not yet clear how it may prevent cancer.

New ways to find cancer faster

Finding breast lumps through manual exams and mammograms may soon be a thing of the past. A two-second test is now available that detects cancers way before any signs of the disease. And early detection may give you valuable time to nip cancer in the bud.

A new saliva test is simpler and less painful than even a blood test, and it may turn out to be more reliable. Researchers in Houston have identified proteins in your saliva that are different in women with breast cancer than in women without — and different from women with only benign breast tumors. If this new technology works, breast cancer could be diagnosed with a simple visit to your dentist. Other technologies in the works may give your doctor even more methods to find breast tumors.

■ Elasticity imaging. This technique may let you skip an invasive biopsy, giving a quick answer to the question of whether a breast lesion is malignant or harmless. It combines a manual exam with scanning to see how tissue in your breast moves when it's pushed. Malignant tumors seem to be stiffer.

■ Digital breast tomosynthesis. The procedure is still being developed, but it may offer a scan that's not as painful as a mammogram, since less pressure is required to get a good image. Another plus is creation of a 3-D picture rather than a flat image.

■ Radar breast imaging. Experts in England are working on a breast scanning machine that uses radio waves. Unlike with a mammogram, you wouldn't be exposed to radiation. This test would also be more comfortable than a mammogram, since it allows your breast to sit in a round ceramic cup rather than being squashed between acrylic sheets.

Take a shot at incontinence relief

Problems with urine leakage may be a part of aging, but they're still embarrassing. If you're willing to brave injections, you have two choices that may help stop the problem.

Collagen injections. This protein works to bulk up tissues when it's injected into the area around the urethra, the tube that takes urine out of your body. The procedure tightens the urethral sphincter and keeps urine from leaking.

Collagen injections are given as a series of two to three shots, at least four weeks apart. In one study, collagen worked for 93 percent of the women who tried it, especially those with stress incontinence who previously had surgery. Collagen may also be a good choice if you're too frail to have the surgery or you don't want a long recovery time.

But as with other treatments that use fillers, collagen injections must be repeated when the bulking agent flattens out — after around a year. Since they cost about $5,000 for a set of shots, they may not be the best choice for younger people who need long-term treatment.

Botox injections. It's better known as a treatment for wrinkles, but injections of botulinum-A neurotoxin can also treat overactive bladder. Botox is injected into the detrusor muscle in the bladder wall, which contracts when you urinate. Injections block the nerves that connect to this muscle to keep it from contracting too often. Botox works for overactive bladder up to 96 percent of the time, and it may be a good choice when anticholinergic drugs haven't done the job.

The downsides to using Botox are cost and uncertainty about long-term effects. A set of injections costs roughly $1,400 and lasts only about seven months. At each treatment, the bladder is injected at 20 to 30 locations. If you need repeated treatments over the years, the shots can cause scar tissue to build up, which could cause problems in the future.

Surprising side effect from common drug

If you have urge incontinence, your doctor may prescribe a drug like Ditropan or Oxytrol (oxybutynin). Both are types of anticholinergics. They work by stopping bladder spasms, allowing your bladder to hold more, and delaying the urge to urinate.

But there is a negative to these drugs. They can get in the way of clear thinking and hamper your ability to carry out basic activities of daily living. People in nursing homes who were taking cholinesterase inhibitors — used to slow mental decline — had even more trouble thinking when they began taking an anticholinergic drug. Wider research confirmed the problem occurred even in people not taking the other drugs. If you start taking medication for incontinence, talk to your doctor about what to expect.

Home test catches cancer early

Don't wait for symptoms if you're at risk for bladder cancer. Try a home test that can find this common cancer early.

The test uses strips that change color when they come into contact with urine that has blood in it. Research shows using the strips lets you find bladder cancer early, when it can be treated. Blood in the urine is the first sign of bladder cancer in 90 percent of cases. But don't panic if you test positive. It can also be a sign of other problems, like kidney stones.

Bladder tumors grow quickly, so if you're at risk, you would need to test frequently. Risk factors include having been previously diagnosed with bladder cancer or having bladder birth defects. Those who smoke or are exposed to certain chemicals at work — like in the dry-cleaning or paper-manufacturing industries — may also be at risk.

You can buy test strips over the counter at a drugstore or online. A pack of 50 strips costs about $30.

5 things you should know about prostate cancer

There's a lot of talk in the news about prostate cancer — what to eat to avoid it, who needs a test, new treatments. Here are the five key facts you need to know about this disease.

Not all men need a test. A PSA (prostate specific antigen) blood test can help identify prostate cancer that may become life threatening in five to 25 years. That's a large time span. But prostate cancer tends to grow so slowly that — even if a PSA test shows you might have cancer — you may die of something else before the prostate cancer is a problem.

For older men, the United States Preventive Services Task Force says screening for prostate cancer does more harm than good. They say you shouldn't get a PSA screening if you are older than age 75 or have less than a 10-year life expectancy because of another health condition. Other men should weigh the possible benefits of the test against its risks, like false alarms that can lead to additional testing and treatment.

Aspirin may affect PSA scores. Don't start aspirin therapy for prostate cancer without talking to your doctor. Aspirin and other nonsteroidal anti-inflammatory drugs (NSAIDs) seem to lower PSA levels, which could be a sign of protection against cancer, or they could simply lower PSA levels without having any effect on prostate cancer development. It's still unknown if NSAIDs reduce prostate cancer risk or artificially lower PSA scores.

Avoid sex before a PSA test. Some studies show ejaculation one or two days before a PSA test may increase PSA levels in the blood, giving falsely high readings. Consequently, men should abstain from sex for 72 hours before a PSA test.

New test may be better than PSA. Look for a simple blood test for early prostate cancer antigen-2 (EPCA-2). It tests for a protein found in prostate cancer cells, and it's more accurate than the PSA test at distinguishing between cancerous and noncancerous prostates. PSA results can also indicate other prostate disorders — not just cancer. Also, EPCA-2 is better at identifying cancers that have begun to spread, so men who need treatment without delay can get it. The test should be available soon.

Targeted treatments save healthy tissue. Focal techniques target only the cancer, sparing healthy tissue. Unlike prostate surgery, these treatments may let you avoid side effects, like incontinence and impotence.

■ Focal cryoablation. Sometimes called a "male lumpectomy," this procedure freezes and removes just the tumor.

■ High-dose-rate brachytherapy, or implanted radioactive seeds. Rather than leaving the seeds in your body for months as in traditional brachytherapy, they're implanted via hollow plastic needles and removed within 24 to 48 hours. It's as effective as traditional brachytherapy, but it causes fewer side effects. Also, since you don't carry the radioactive seeds around for long, you don't risk affecting family members with radiation.

■ MRI-guided brachytherapy. This refinement allows the seeds to be placed more accurately for better treatment.

Eyes & ears: a lifetime warranty

Delicious ways to save your sight

Some foods seem specially designed to preserve your vision, thanks to powerful natural compounds known as antioxidants.

Rockin' rooibos tea. Keep your eyesight keen as you age with this fragrant tea loaded with vision-protecting nutrients. It's not green or black. It's red. The antioxidants in this African tea can help prevent diabetic complications, including diabetic cataracts and retinopathy.

In diabetes, your body pumps out loads of harmful substances called free radicals — so many, in fact, that they overwhelm your natural defenses. Antioxidant-rich foods and beverages like red rooibos tea shore up those defenses, helping prevent and treat the oxidative damage these compounds cause. The antioxidants in this tasty tea may even guard against age-related macular degeneration (AMD).

Look for it in your local supermarket. It brews just like a normal tea. Steep the leaves anywhere from five to 10 minutes. The longer you steep it in very hot water, the more antioxidants you get.

Clever little kiwi. The famous Blue Mountains Eye Study followed nearly 2,500 people for more than 10 years and discovered that those who got the most vitamin C were about half as likely to develop nuclear cataracts.

Once again, you can probably blame free radicals. Everyday cell work produces some free radicals; others are caused by the sun's ultraviolet (UV) rays striking your eyes. Either way, these compounds can do real damage, and the lenses of your eyes are especially vulnerable. Damage done here may speed up the development of cataracts.

Your eyes, especially the lenses, contain lots of vitamin C. This vitamin plays a vital role here, absorbing UV radiation and neutralizing free radicals before they do harm. Folks in the Blue Mountains Eye Study got an average of 500 milligrams (mg) of vitamin C daily, mainly from cruciferous vegetables, potatoes, citrus fruits, and fruit juice.

One kiwi boasts 84 mg of vitamin C, getting you off on the right foot. If kiwis aren't your thing, consider orange juice. Researchers say fruit juice may offer a more concentrated source of C than whole fruit.

Sassy yellow spice. Turmeric, the yellow spice in curry powder, may head off diabetic retinopathy, another disease linked to the oxidative damage done by free radicals.

Turmeric packs a secret weapon — the compound curcumin, which gives the spice its yellow color. A rat study showed curcumin helped block oxidative stress and inflammation, two of the factors behind diabetic retinopathy. This leads researchers to believe it could do the same thing in people, either slowing or preventing the development of this eye disease.

As an antioxidant, curcumin is 10 times better than vitamin E at nixing free radicals. Although it's not a cure on its own, it may prove helpful alongside other treatments for controlling the complications of diabetes.

The vital vision shopping list

Head to the grocery store with this list in hand, and keep your eyesight sharp into your 90s. Eating the foods listed here could cut your risk of degenerative eye diseases, such as age-related macular degeneration, in half.

Salmon. Older eyes can be sharp eyes. Just make sure you eat fatty fish twice weekly. Fish are swimming in omega-3 fatty acids, two of which may stop age-related macular degeneration (AMD) from getting worse. People with early-stage wet or dry AMD who got the most DHA and EPA omega-3s were least likely to see their disease advance.

The cells in your eyes that sense light die off in this and other degenerative eye diseases. These and other eye cells need DHA to make NPD1, a compound that squashes inflammation and protects them from dying. Experts say just two to three servings of fatty fish, such as salmon, tuna, mackerel, or herring, each week should give you all the DHA and EPA you need to beat this eye disease.

Whole wheat bread. DHA and EPA offer the most protection if you eat them in combination with a low-glycemic index (GI) diet full of foods such as whole grains. The Blue Mountains Eye Study agrees. Over 10 years, people who ate mostly low-GI breads and cereals, such as oatmeal, and got plenty of cereal fiber were one-third less likely to develop AMD. A diet loaded with high-GI foods, on the other hand, boosted people's risk of this blinding disease an incredible 77 percent.

High-GI foods make your blood sugar rise rapidly, and a quick spike may damage cells in your retina. Low-GI foods, on the other hand, release their sugar into your bloodstream gradually, avoiding those sharp spikes. Simply swapping five slices of white bread for whole wheat every day could prevent 8 percent of advanced AMD cases over the next five years. Substitute whole grains for refined ones in your own diet, and you could be one of the lucky.

Chicken. Australians who ate 10 or more servings of red meat weekly were 50 percent more likely to get AMD. But Australians who ate chicken at least three times a week cut their risk in half.

Try broadening the protein you eat during the week. Enjoy red meat sparingly, and focus instead on poultry and fish.

Low-fat milk. Vitamin D may prevent you from getting AMD. A new study found that people with the highest blood levels of this vitamin were one-third less likely to have early-stage AMD. Milk was linked to a lower risk, too.

Scientists think vitamin D packs a one-two punch. It may douse the inflammation that contributes to AMD, plus prevent the growth of rogue blood vessels that are the hallmark of wet AMD.

Fishy end to dry eyes

You are what you eat, and eating more fatty fish like tuna or salmon may ward off dry eyes. Women who ate tuna fish five or more times a week were nearly 70 percent less likely to have dry eye syndrome, compared to those who only ate it once a week.

Certain compounds in your body stir up inflammation, which in turn plays a starring role in dry eye syndrome. Fatty fish are awash in two omega-3 fatty acids, DHA and EPA, which douse the flames of these inflammatory compounds.

Stay 20/20 with spinach

Popeye must have had perfect vision with all the spinach he ate. Green leafy goodies like spinach and kale are chock full of two sight-saving antioxidants named lutein and zeaxanthin.

Attack AMD. The cells in your eyes naturally churn out a compound called A2E as a byproduct of all their sight-seeing activity.

Unfortunately, the light entering your eyes causes oxidative stress, which in turn throws a wrench in how your cells handle A2E.

Under this kind of stress, A2E jams up the mitochondria, tiny power plants inside cells, so they can't pump out enough fuel. Without enough energy, cleaning and maintenance fall by the wayside. In turn, A2E buildup gets worse, like trash that doesn't get taken out. Eventually, important vision cells start dying — and your body doesn't replace them.

Lab studies now show that certain antioxidants could completely counteract the ravages of oxidative stress, putting a stop to this vicious cycle. Lutein and zeaxanthin seem especially potent. They absorb blue light as it enters your eyes and keep it from reaching and damaging the cells needed for sight.

An Australian study found that people who ate the most lutein and zeaxanthin from food were amazingly two-thirds less likely to develop age-related macular degeneration (AMD). Even people who ate an average amount dropped their risk by one-third. Start building your meals around green leafy vegetables, and enjoy your eyesight into old age.

Cancel out cataracts. The protection doesn't stop there, though. Out of more than 35,000 women, those who ate the most lutein and zeaxanthin were 18 percent less likely to develop cataracts. Some of the same reasons apply here, too. By filtering out blue light, lutein and zeaxanthin help prevent oxidative damage in delicate eye tissue.

Duck diabetic retinopathy. These compounds combat diabetic retinopathy, too, by nixing inflammation, growth factors, and damaging free radicals that all contribute to this disease. While the combination of these two antioxidants didn't lower blood sugar in animal studies, it did prevent retinal damage from getting worse.

Researchers think the same could prove true for humans, and that loading up on foods rich in these compounds could put the brakes on diabetic retinopathy, or help prevent it in the first place.

Other natural remedies

Keep hearing keen into old age

Going deaf doesn't have to be part of growing older. These nutritional supplements may both improve the hearing you have and preserve it into the future.

Sharpen your hearing. A common B vitamin could help save your hearing. Dutch researchers studied people ages 50 to 70 who were beginning to lose their hearing. Half took 800 milligrams (mg) of folic acid a day, while the other half took a placebo, or fake pill. After three years of treatment, the placebo group had lost more hearing than the vitamin group. The difference was small, but every little bit counts.

Food in the Netherlands is not fortified with folic acid as it is in the United States. Experts don't know if getting more of this vitamin via supplements will give your hearing an additional edge if you already get plenty from fortified foods. Talk to your doctor before taking the plunge, especially if you use blood-thinning medications.

Guard against noise. A combination supplement containing magnesium, beta carotene, and vitamins C and E may shield your ears from noise-related hearing loss. Scientists used to think that the intense vibrations from loud noises damaged your inner ear, leading to hearing loss. Now they believe the process is more complex and, possibly, preventable.

When loud noise enters your ears, free radicals form harmful compounds that can destroy the tiny cells in your inner ear. You may lose some hearing temporarily but regain it later. Over time, though, the damage becomes permanent. Animal research shows a supplement cocktail made with these nutrients could prevent noise-related hearing damage if taken before exposure to loud noise.

Magnesium speeds up healing by improving blood flow to your inner ear, while the others act as powerful antioxidants, nixing those free radicals before they harm your hearing cells. Together, these nutrients could help protect against both noise- and age-related hearing loss. The company OTOMedicine will begin selling this supplement under the name Auraquell once the FDA approves it.

Silence the din of tinnitus

Coenzyme Q10 could help quiet the constant ringing or roaring in your ears. A small, four-month study found the supplement improved tinnitus in people who had low blood levels of CoQ10 in their bodies. It didn't, however, help people who already had normal CoQ10 levels.

Safe supplements keep vision sharp

Age-related macular degeneration (AMD) has no cure, but growing evidence suggests certain supplements can prevent it or slow its progress.

B's are key. They've long been known to guard heart health, but researchers discovered that B vitamins can defend vision, too. Women at high risk for heart disease were given a B-complex supplement containing:

- 50 milligrams (mg) of B6

- 2.5 mg of folic acid

- 1 mg of B12

After seven years, researchers discovered these women were 35 to 40 percent less likely to get AMD than those not on vitamins. The protection kicked in after only two years of treatment.

Experts suspect a link between high levels of homocysteine — a compound that raises your risk for heart disease and hardening of the arteries — and the eye disease AMD. The three B vitamins used here lower homocysteine and may work as antioxidants, counteracting free radical damage and boosting blood vessel function in your eyes.

Consider a B-vitamin-complex supplement if you suffer from heart disease or are at high risk for it. Heart-related conditions may make you more likely to develop AMD.

Vitamin combos show promise. Made famous by the Age-Related Eye Disease Study (AREDS), this combination supplement taken four times a day slowed the progression of AMD and preserved vision sharpness in people with the disease. It contained:

- 7160 international units (IU) of vitamin A as beta carotene

- 113 mg of vitamin C

- 100 IU of vitamin E

- 17.4 mg of zinc

- 0.4 mg of copper

The same formula is now available over the counter as Ocuvite Preser-Vision and a delayed-release form called ICAPS. A third product, Natural Vision Care, contains some of the same ingredients, but in smaller amounts, along with the antioxidants lutein and zeaxanthin. All three products passed recent quality tests by an independent lab.

A new combination supplement may one day hit the market for AMD. The Carotenoids in Age-Related Maculopathy (CARMA) Study is currently testing a mixture of lutein, zeaxanthin, zinc, and vitamins C and E. If it works, you may soon see it on store shelves as well.

Healthful living

Get moving to keep eyes keen

Don your sneakers and grab the dog. Going for a daily run will help preserve your vision and ward off three of the most serious sight problems.

Cataracts. They're the most common cause of blindness, making them a top priority for prevention. Researchers tailed runners for seven years, tracking their health changes as part of the National Runners' Health Study. Men who ran more than 5.7 miles a day slashed their cataract risk by more than one-third compared to men who ran less than 1.4 miles daily. Speed counts, too. Men who ran the fastest halved their risk, compared to the slowest, or "least fit," runners.

Your heart and lung health appears to be the key, and running keeps these organs in tip-top shape. No need to start training for a marathon, though. Experts say simply walking may also knock down your cataract risk.

Macular degeneration. Having fleet feet can help you beat the odds against age-related macular degeneration (AMD). It strikes one out of every four people over the age of 75, but running can reduce your risk. For every 0.6 mile (1 kilometer) people ran every day, their chances of AMD dropped 10 percent. People who ran between 1.2 and 2.5 miles each day cut their risk 19 percent. Those who ran more slashed their risk nearly in half.

Glaucoma. A little aerobic exercise, such as running for 30 minutes, can lower pressure inside your eye. That's a boon because elevated eye pressure can lead to glaucoma.

Not all exercise helps, though. Lifting weights can actually make you more likely to develop or worsen glaucoma. Weight-lifting exercises like bench presses can temporarily increase the pressure in your eyes, especially if you hold your breath while lifting. Frequent changes in eye pressure like this have been linked to glaucoma down the road.

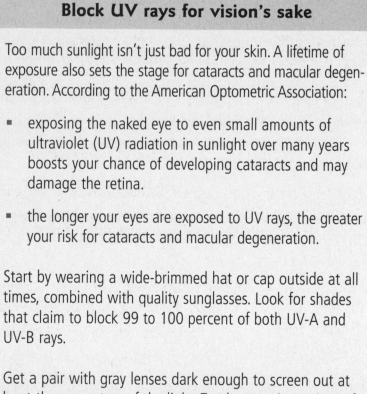

Block UV rays for vision's sake

Too much sunlight isn't just bad for your skin. A lifetime of exposure also sets the stage for cataracts and macular degeneration. According to the American Optometric Association:

- exposing the naked eye to even small amounts of ultraviolet (UV) radiation in sunlight over many years boosts your chance of developing cataracts and may damage the retina.

- the longer your eyes are exposed to UV rays, the greater your risk for cataracts and macular degeneration.

Start by wearing a wide-brimmed hat or cap outside at all times, combined with quality sunglasses. Look for shades that claim to block 99 to 100 percent of both UV-A and UV-B rays.

Get a pair with gray lenses dark enough to screen out at least three-quarters of the light. Try them on in a mirror. If you can easily see your eyes through the lenses, they probably aren't dark enough.

Defend ears from everyday dangers

Swinging titanium rather than steel golf clubs can actually lead to hearing loss. It's called "impact noise," and a new study shows that thin-faced titanium clubs make a much louder smacking sound than the old-fashioned steel kind.

Sounds louder than 85 decibels (dB) jeopardize your hearing. Chronic exposure to loud noise damages the delicate hair-like cells in your inner ear, which are key to the whole process of hearing. The damage accumulates over time and, unfortunately, seems to be permanent.

Golf clubs aren't the only hidden dangers, however. Beware of high-tech threats in the form of headphones and personal music players such as iPods and MP3 players. The maximum volume on an iPod is more than 100 dB when using the Apple earbuds that come with the device. At that level, you could damage your hearing in minutes.

The same holds true for other devices and headphones. At full volume, most are only safe to listen to for:

- 18 minutes with foam earphones that fit over your ears.

- five minutes for regular earphones that fit inside your ears.

- three minutes for special "isolator" earphones designed to block outside noise.

Play it safe. Limit the amount of time you listen to a personal music player, and never set the volume higher than 70 percent of the maximum. Some devices, like iPods, allow you to set your own maximum-volume limits.

Guard your ears. Wear earplugs or other protection when golfing, riding a lawnmower, using a power saw, attending arena sporting events, or doing other loud activities — including riding public transportation. A New York City study found that the sound levels inside subway cars and on platforms exceeded what is safe.

Give smart gifts. Remember, hearing loss starts early. When buying toys for the little ones in your life, pay attention to how much sound they make. The Sight & Hearing Association discovered that 14 out of 18 toys tested were louder than 100 dB, enough to damage a tot's hearing in 15 minutes. Even "safe" ones can harm a child's hearing if held against their ear.

Play it safe with cell phones

Spending too much time on a cell phone could damage your hearing. Over the long term, using a cell phone for more than an hour a day led to high-frequency hearing loss, usually in people's phone ear.

Blame cell phone radiation, not loud-talking family and friends. Phones that use GSM technology put out electromagnetic radiation that can interfere with the activity of cells in your ear.

Pay attention to symptoms like ringing, warmth, or fullness in your ears while on the phone. These signs suggest you may be losing your hearing. Try to spend less than an hour a day on the cell phone. Use a landline phone, if you have one, for longer calls.

Tame tinnitus with proven treatments

The whooshing, ringing, hissing, or roaring in your ears can rob you of every quiet moment in life if you let it. These treatments can help rescue them again.

Take care of TMJ. Temporomandibular joint (TMJ) disorders involve the main joint in your jaw and often go hand in hand with tinnitus. Your jaw muscles and nerves are closely connected to the ones in your ear, so TMJ problems can interfere with the hearing process, causing tinnitus.

Treating one condition may soothe the other. Headaches, bite problems, a locked jaw, clicking noises, and ear pain are all signs of a jaw disorder. Treating a TMJ issue will most likely help your tinnitus if:

■ both problems began around the same time.

■ they tend to act up at the same time.

■ both conditions worsen when you are under stress.

Soothe it with sound therapy. Adding background noise can cover, or mask, tinnitus, making it less noticeable, loud, and bothersome. Creating soothing sounds can be as simple as turning on a table fan at night or as high-tech as wearing an in-ear device similar to a hearing aid. Sound machines that offer backdrops ranging from ocean waves to white noise may help, too.

Don't rely on sound alone, however. This therapy works best if you combine it with counseling, rather than use it on its own.

See a professional. Counseling can go a long way toward maintaining your sanity while living with tinnitus. One type, called cognitive therapy, tries to change how you emotionally react to the noise, rather than cure the ringing itself. The therapist will tailor the program specifically to you. Counseling generally works best alongside other tinnitus treatments, such as sound therapy or medication.

Stop the stress loop. Relaxation techniques such as biofeedback can help you learn to control otherwise automatic physical reactions, including your pulse rate, muscle tension, and skin temperature. The idea is to manage stress better and change how your body reacts to it.

Get needled. Several small studies suggest acupuncture can ease, if not cure, tinnitus. The most important acupuncture spots are on your head, about 1.75 inches above each ear. Experts think this ancient technique may quiet the crazy nerve signals traveling from the ear to your brain and help the ear work normally again.

Dodge these triggers. Try to avoid alcohol, nicotine, caffeine, and stressful situations. All can aggravate the clamor in your ears.

---

eMedical alternatives

When hearing loss can be cured

Not all hearing loss is permanent. For instance, conductive hearing loss, where something blocks sound waves from reaching your inner ear, can often be reversed. Fluid in the ear, earwax buildup, or a punctured eardrum are all treatable.

Medications can cause problems, too. High doses of aspirin and other salicylates can trigger tinnitus and hearing loss. So can non-steroidal anti-inflammatory drugs (NSAIDs), including ibuprofen and naproxen, in high doses or with long-term use. Luckily, hearing usually returns to normal when you stop taking them.

That's not the case with all drugs, though. Some, like these, can lead to permanent hearing loss.

- a class of antibiotics known as aminoglycosides, including gentamicin, streptomycin, and kanamycin, especially when given intravenously

- in adults over age 53, high doses of the antibiotic vancomycin, used to treat MRSA infections

- combination hormone replacement therapy containing estrogen and progestin, which can accelerate age-related hearing loss

- loop diuretics, including bumetanide (Bumex), ethacrynic acid (Edecrin), furosemide (Lasix), and torsemide (Demadex)

- anti-cancer drugs known as anti-neoplastics, such as cisplatin and carboplatin

See your doctor immediately if you develop hearing problems while on these medications, but don't stop taking them on your own.

Guide to selecting a safe device

You get what you pay for, and scrimping on a cheap hearing aid can actually hasten hearing loss. You may see these devices sold for hunting, or hearing bird songs, whispered speech, and distant sound. But one thing they're not — a hearing aid.

A new study tested eight over-the-counter hearing devices sold for under $100 and three between $100 and $500. Researchers discovered that, not only did the cheap devices work poorly, particularly in settings with background noise like restaurants — they may harm what is left of your hearing.

Across the board, the cheap devices over-magnified low-frequency sounds and failed to magnify high-frequency ones. This makes them pointless as hearing aids, since most hearing loss happens in the high-frequency range. Add to that, they magnified some sounds so much they could damage your hearing.

"Aside from being of extremely poor quality, very-low-cost hearing aids — those under $100 — have the potential to damage your hearing because they send very loud sounds into the ear," says Copenhagen University researcher Susanna Love Callaway. Mid-priced devices fared better. "The study's mid-range hearing aids were of higher quality and were not considered a safety hazard."

Before you buy one, though, you still need to see an audiologist, or hearing expert. Not all hearing loss is the same, and different aids work better for different types of loss. An audiologist can test your hearing, help you choose the best device for your type, and even fit you with it. "Based on the research, the best advice for consumers is to talk to an audiologist. Because hearing aids have complex technical features, they need to be fitted and customized to the individual," says the study's co-author Jerry Punch, a professor in Michigan State University's Department of Communicative Sciences and Disorders.

Of course, people turn to cheap hearing devices in the first place partly because Medicare won't pay for them. However, some Medicare Advantage plans will. Think ahead. If you know you need a hearing aid, start researching policies and coverage. Ask questions, and find out which will cover hearing aids. If you already have a Medicare Advantage policy, call your provider and ask if hearing aids are covered. You may be pleasantly surprised.

Overlooked hearing aid hazard

Getting an MRI could short-circuit your hearing if you wear a cochlear implant (CI). MRIs produce strong magnetic fields that can demagnetize the magnet in your CI.

Tell the MRI technician if you have a CI with a non-removable magnet. Don't get into a 3.0T MRI machine set up for routine scans. Instead, have the technician adjust the scanner so that the angle between the MRI magnet and your CI magnet is less than 80 degrees. This will help protect both you and your implant.

New hope for tinnitus treatment

Don't believe that nothing can help your tinnitus. Too many people get told this when, in fact, promising new treatments can help improve, even cure, this disorder.

Silence the sound with hearing aids. If you suffer from tinnitus, you probably have some hearing loss as well. The odds are in your favor. Tinnitus improves in three out of five people who use a hearing aid, and one in five gets major relief. These devices offer two big benefits.

- Hearing the outside sounds around you helps you tune out the ringing in your ears. The very act of listening to something other than your tinnitus actually exercises the auditory part of your brain. Experts say this, in turn, may block your brain's ability to hear the ringing. Eventually, your brain relegates it to background noise and tunes it out.

- Improving your hearing can reduce stress, not to mention allow you to communicate better. As a result, the tinnitus becomes easier to cope with.

Programmable digital hearing aids did more for tinnitus in one study than did older analogue models. Ask your doctor or audiologist whether a hearing aid could help you.

Tickle your brain. It has a long, strange name, but research suggests transcranial magnetic stimulation (TMS) may soothe tinnitus symptoms in some people.

This disorder doesn't affect just your ears. It's linked to real, physical changes in your brain and nervous system. TMS sends low-frequency magnetic stimulation to the part of your brain that processes sound. This creates a small magnetic field that quiets down some of these brain cells, reducing or eliminating the noise.

The tinnitus tends to return within a week or two, but getting a maintenance dose of TMS when your symptoms start coming back may keep it quiet longer. Not everyone with the condition responds to TMS treatment, but about half do get relief.

Ask about medicines. No medicines can currently treat tinnitus, but that may soon change. A new drug now under testing may cure tinnitus caused by ear-damaging loud noise or medications.

Scientists think tinnitus occurs when something goes wrong with the receptors on hearing cells, making your brain "hear" sounds that don't exist. The new drug, AM-101, blocks those broken receptors so they stop sending fake noise signals to your brain. In theory, the clamor stops, too.

First, a doctor numbs your eardrum with a local anesthetic, then injects the drug directly through the eardrum into your middle ear. So far, scientists have only tested AM-101 in people who recently developed tinnitus. They aren't sure the drug will help those who have lived with it for a long time. More research is necessary. In the meantime, stay tuned for more treatments to help you live a life beyond this disorder.

Tips for finding a trouble-free phone

Cell phones work with hearing devices better than ever, and finding the right one just got easier. The Federal Communications Commission now requires cell phones to work better with hearing aids and cochlear implants. You should get less static and interference and enjoy a better telecoil connection.

Not all phones are hearing aid compatible (HAC), but it's easy to find one that is. Look for the HAC label on the phone's package, in its user manual, or on the information card next to the in-store display. If you can't find a label, it's not compatible. For cell phones that are HAC, look for one:

- rated T3 or T4 if your cochlear implant or hearing aid uses a telecoil.

- rated M3 or M4 if your hearing aid has a microphone.

- that lets you control the lighting on the keypad and display, which can interfere with telecoils.

- that vibrates or flashes when a call comes in.

- with a speaker phone option, so you can hold the phone farther away to cut down on hearing aid interference.

■ with connections for assistive devices, such as TTY.

Try out several different phones before buying one, and ask about the cancellation and return policies before you sign any contracts.

Better tests catch eye diseases early

An ounce of prevention is worth a pound of cure, but catching an eye disease early is almost as good. That's why eye exams for blinding diseases like macular degeneration and glaucoma are crucial to keeping your vision keen. New tests can catch these diseases earlier than ever, and with minimum discomfort.

Spot AMD. Recent advances may make screenings for age-related macular degeneration (AMD) easier and more accurate. A single gene boosts your risk of this disease an incredible 700 percent, and a simple blood test can detect it. People who learn they have the AMD gene can act early to drop their risk through diet and lifestyle changes, before they develop the disease. Experts urge people with a family history of AMD to ask about getting tested. A separate test helps doctors figure out which people with dry AMD will lose their vision. Not everyone does, but until now experts couldn't predict who would. The new exam predicts vision loss by having you read under low lighting conditions. Knowing your odds can help you plan for the future, if you have AMD.

Stay one step ahead of glaucoma. Get your eyes checked every two years if your brother or sister has glaucoma, even if the first exam turns out normal. First-degree relatives of people with the condition have a higher-than-average chance of developing it themselves. Siblings of someone with glaucoma face an even greater risk — four times higher than the normal population.

A new device may make the glaucoma test easier to take and the results more accurate. The standard visual field test is uncomfortable, awkward, and not always correct. The new screener, called Virtual Perimetry (VIP), looks like a pair of goggles, is easier to wear, and gives fewer false results. Researchers at Tel Aviv University are still perfecting the device, but expect to see it soon in the United States.

Dodge diabetic retinopathy. An ouch-free test may replace the old, unpleasant one. Fluorescein angiography, the standard test for diabetic retinopathy, involves getting a shot containing dye, then taking a series of photographs of your eyes, looking for abnormalities.

Too many people put off the test to avoid the shot. The new exam doesn't rely on dye, however. It uses a laser to safely map your retina — no injections necessary. It may one day also replace fluorescein angiography in diagnosing AMD and other vascular eye diseases.

Surprising source of vision problems

Your cholesterol medication could be to blame for some vision problems. It's rare, but research links statin drugs to double vision, droopy upper eyelids, and loss of full range of motion in the eyes, even at regular doses.

Call your doctor if any of these symptoms appear. She can switch you to a different cholesterol drug, which should make these vision problems fade away.

---

3 things to know before cataract surgery

Gone are the days when you only had one type of cataract lens to choose from. New ones can correct everything from astigmatism to nearsightedness.

Consider the choices. Conventional cataract lens implants are monofocal, meaning you can only focus on near or far distances in the affected eye, and you'll probably still have to wear glasses to compensate.

New, multifocal lenses offer more options. They're better at correcting near-vision than monofocals, and nine out of 10 people who get them don't need glasses afterward. Special toric lenses, on the other hand, can correct astigmatism.

People who choose multifocal lenses see the best results if they get them in both eyes. The AcrySof ReSTOR and ReZoom brands seem to have fewer side effects, such as nighttime glare and halos.

Unfortunately, Medicare typically won't pay more for these specialty lenses. It will, however, cover them up to the cost of conventional lenses. You'll pay the additional expense out of pocket.

Rethink lens replacement. Take your time when deciding whether to have surgery. New glasses, brighter lighting, anti-glare sunglasses, or a magnifying glass can go a long way in overcoming early cataract symptoms. Experts say you only need to have a cataract removed if it interferes with daily activities, such as driving, reading, or watching television. In most cases, delaying surgery won't result in long-term eye damage or make the operation more difficult.

Avoid complications. Tell your eye doctor if you take an alpha-blocker such as tamsulosin (Flomax). These drugs typically treat an enlarged prostate, but they can also complicate cataract surgery if your doctor doesn't know you take them. Flomax has been linked to more post-op complications, but other alpha-blockers can cause problems, too.

These medications affect the iris of your eye, making it contract during surgery. That's a problem, because the iris must stay dilated, or open, for the surgeon to remove and replace the cataract lens behind it.

You can still undergo cataract surgery. Simply tell your surgeon beforehand if you take these drugs, or if you used to take them. Don't stop taking them on your own.

Stay 'focused' with free eye exams

There is no reason to let your eyesight fail when you can get eye exams free through EyeCare America, the American Academy of Ophthalmology's public service program.

Around the country, ophthalmologists volunteer their time to give free exams, and in some cases treatment, to people in need. Through EyeCare America, you can get screened for glaucoma, age-related macular degeneration (AMD), and diabetic eye diseases including diabetic retinopathy, among other vision problems.

You must meet certain criteria to qualify for a free exam. The qualifications vary based on which type of screening you need, but generally you must:

- be a United States citizen or legal resident

- not have had a recent eye exam

- not have coverage from an HMO or the Veterans Administration

For a diabetes or AMD eye exam, you must be over the age of 65. For a glaucoma test, you must be at particular risk for it, based on your family history, age, or race.

EyeCare America accepts Medicare or insurance reimbursement as payment, with no out-of-pocket cost to you. The exam is free even if you have no insurance coverage. Call 800-222-EYES (3937) to find out if you qualify.

Say goodbye to irritating eye drops

High-tech contacts could make eye drops and drugs a thing of the past. Researchers have found a way to embed medicine directly into contact lenses, delivering the drug straight to the eye for more than four weeks at a time. The new lenses are still in the testing stages, but keep an eye out for them in the future.

7

Anti-aging tactics for teeth & gums

Top-notch brews for healthy teeth

No need to toss out your coffee pot or give up tea to save your teeth. The very beverages you love can actually help prevent cavities, gum disease, dry mouth, and oral cancer — cancers of the mouth and throat.

Fight cavities. Coffee as well as black, green, and oolong teas are chock-full of cavity-blasting antioxidants called polyphenols. These natural plant chemicals act as antibacterial agents and keep cavity-causing bacteria from clinging to your teeth.

Unlike soda and orange juice, coffee and tea won't damage tooth enamel. They do, however, tend to stain your teeth. To avoid staining, drink cold teas through a straw. For other beverages, rinse your mouth with water after drinking, then brush your teeth 30 minutes later.

Battle gum disease. A Japanese study found that men who drank the most green tea had healthier gums and a lower risk of periodontal disease, which attacks gums and the bones supporting your teeth.

The polyphenols in green tea block disease-causing organisms from setting up house in your mouth, plus reduce inflammation.

Experts think polyphenols interfere with your body's inflammatory response to mouth bacteria, which may actually help keep your mouth healthy. What's good for your gums may prove good for your heart and blood sugar, too, since gum inflammation has been linked to heart disease and diabetes.

Soothe Sjogren's syndrome. Out-of-control inflammation in your tear and salivary glands mark this autoimmune disease. Eventually, these glands stop working, leading to eye and mouth problems. There's no known cure, but the polyphenols in green tea may help.

Mice with Sjogren-like symptoms drank water laced with a green tea polyphenol. After four months, mice getting this brew had less inflammation and damage to their salivary glands than Sjogren mice drinking just water. Researchers suspect the brew could help prevent or manage this disease in people, too.

Avoid oral cancer. Drinking coffee could help you dodge oral cancers. In a Japanese study of nearly 40,000 people, those who drank at least one cup of coffee daily had half the risk of oral, pharyngeal, and esophageal cancers. Even people normally prone to these cancers, such as those who smoked or drank alcohol, gained protection from coffee.

Smooth treat saves choppers

A scoop of creamy yogurt every day may guard your mouth against periodontitis. This condition can lead to loose teeth, receding gums, inflammation, and the breakdown of your gums, teeth, and bones that support your teeth. People who ate at least one-quarter cup of yogurt daily had a healthier mouth and were 50 to 60 percent less likely to have periodontitis.

Make your mouth happy with little red fruits

Cavities, gum disease, and gingivitis should have you seeing red — in the form of cranberries and pomegranates.

Cranberry to the rescue. Cranberry compounds could put a stop to cavities, gum disease, and gingivitis. The plaque that forms on teeth harbors bacteria, which in turn feed into these mouth problems. Cranberry compounds prevent:

- bad bacteria from sticking to your teeth.

- gum-disease causing bacteria from congregating and setting up house in your mouth.

- your body from overreacting to bacterial invasions and pumping out inflammatory compounds, which tend to worsen the situation and set the stage for gum disease.

Don't rush to the store to stock up on cranberry juice. It's typically too sugary and acidic to do your mouth good. Look for cranberry-infused mouthwashes and toothpastes in the future.

Praise for pomegranate. In a lab study, pure, 100-percent pomegranate juice killed the common, cavity-causing bacteria *Streptococcus mutans*. Eventually, researchers want to add pomegranate compounds to toothpaste and mouthwash to boost their antibacterial power. For now, you can make this fruit juice part of your daily routine.

Steer clear of enamel-eroding foods

You know sodas and sugary candies can eat away your teeth, but so can your favorite canned tea and after-exercise sports drink. The acids in these beverages get most of the blame, but flavor additives do their fair share of damage.

Sports drinks. Drinking these "thirst-quenchers" long term can erode teeth and make them more sensitive. That's because their citric acid eats away at the enamel coating your teeth, then starts to weaken and soften the bone-like material underneath. This can lead to severe damage and eventually tooth loss. As if that's not enough, Gatorade and Powerade drinks also stained teeth in one study.

Sour candies. It's not just the sugar that causes problems. Sour candies get their pucker from citric acid, the most erosive kind of acid in your diet. Tests found that most sour candies were more acidic than sodas. In fact, Warheads Sour Spray liquid and Altoids Citrus Sours hard candy were almost as strong as battery acid. Lemon-, cherry-, and grape-flavored sour sweets are hardest on teeth. Watch out, in particular, for chewy "gummy" candies, powdered candies, sprays, powder-coated gums, and thick, sticky gel candies.

Canned teas and sodas. Besides acids, these drinks boast flavor additives that attach to teeth and aggressively eat away at enamel. Root beer is the safest soda, so choose this if you can't break the carbonated habit. Brew a fresh pot of green or black tea rather than cracking open a prepackaged can or bottle of tea.

You don't have to give up all of your favorite drinks and sweets. Simply snack smartly. These tips can help you enjoy treats while protecting your teeth.

- Eat erosive snacks like sodas, sour candies, and carb-heavy crackers, cookies, and chips with a meal instead of between meals. The extra saliva will buffer their acid and wash them out of your mouth faster.

- Follow your meal with a neutral or slightly alkaline food, such as cheese or milk. You can also try sugar-free gum or sugar-free chewable antacids.

- Don't brush your teeth immediately after eating or drinking something erosive. Acids soften tooth enamel, and toothpaste's abrasiveness can worsen the erosion. Instead, rinse your mouth with water. Wait 30 minutes before brushing to let the enamel re-harden.

- Drink unsweetened tea and water instead of sodas and canned teas. Tea naturally contains fluoride, which helps strengthen tooth enamel. Water can help flush food particles from your mouth and dilute sugars and acids.

- Use the less-abrasive toothpastes made for sensitive teeth rather than the more abrasive whitening toothpastes. If you drink sports drinks regularly, ask your dentist if you should use a special acid-neutralizing, remineralizing toothpaste.

Amazing sweetener fights tooth decay

Not all gummy candies are hard on teeth. Adding the sweetener xylitol to gums and candies can protect your pearly whites from tooth decay. Even the Army has caught on. The U.S. Army began including xylitol-sweetened chewing gum in troops' rations to improve their oral health while on deployment.

Can't chew gum? Look for xylitol-sweetened gummy candies. A study in children showed eating gummy bear candies sweetened with xylitol three times a day cut the number of cavity-causing bacteria lurking in the kids' mouths.

Cheese, chicken, and nuts help guard tooth enamel, too, either by neutralizing acids in your mouth or by providing calcium and phosphorous that remineralize your teeth.

Wise way to beat cancer

You are what you eat. Out of almost half a million people, those who ate the most of these fruits and veggies were least likely to get head and neck cancers, which include cancers of the mouth, nose, sinuses, salivary glands, throat, and lymph nodes in the neck.

- Dried beans, string beans, and peas dropped the risk 20 percent.

- Apples, peaches, nectarines, plums, pears, and strawberries sliced it 40 percent.

- Peppers and tomatoes cut it 18 percent.

■ Carrots shaved it 27 percent.

Vegetables seem especially important in preventing cancer relapse and death. In people with mouth and throat cancers, loading up on vegetables before and after diagnosis was linked to a lower rate of cancer recurrence and longer survival time after diagnosis.

Healthful living

Best brush for cleaning your teeth

Ditching a manual toothbrush could keep your teeth cleaner. A study pitting a manual toothbrush against a power brush found that the power brush used in the study cleaned plaque from teeth 45 percent better. Not only were people's teeth cleaner after brushing, but they also showed less plaque buildup later in the day.

There's more than one type of power brush, and each cleans differently.

■ Counter oscillating brushes use tufts of bristles rotating in opposite directions.

■ Rotating oscillating brushes spin the brush head in one direction, then the other.

■ Ultrasonic brushes use bristles that vibrate at ultrasonic frequencies.

■ Ionic brushes give an electrical charge to the surface of teeth to prevent plaque from sticking.

One power brush seems to rise above the rest. In a review of 42 studies, only rotating oscillating power brushes cleaned better than manual toothbrushes. They consistently did a better job of cutting plaque and preventing gingivitis, or gum inflammation, and reduced gum bleeding.

You don't need a fancy toothbrush to prevent tooth decay. The important thing is to brush regularly with a fluoride toothpaste to remove plaque. Plaque is the main cause of gingivitis and contributes to development of periodontitis, a gum disease marked by inflammation and the breakdown of gums, teeth, and bone.

The American Dental Association (ADA) says people who have trouble using a manual toothbrush may especially benefit from a power brush. No matter which type you choose, pick one that fits comfortably inside your mouth, so it can reach all of your teeth. Look for a brush sporting the ADA's Seal of Acceptance and, if it's a power brush, one certified by Underwriters Laboratories (UL).

Dodge hidden danger of mouthwash

People who use mouthwash may be more likely to get oral cancer, according to new research. Experts know that drinking alcohol and smoking boost your risk of oral cancer, but some studies suggest swishing with an alcohol-containing mouthwash does, too.

Alcohol in drinks makes the cells in your mouth more susceptible to carcinogens, or cancer-causing compounds. But the ethanol used in mouthwash is not the same as the alcohol in beverages. Unlike regular alcohol, ethanol is not a known carcinogen.

Still, new research found that alcohol-containing mouthwashes may have a similar effect. The risk seems small, but the American Dental Association (ADA) recommends playing it safe. The ADA suggests that people with a higher-than-average risk for oral cancers, thanks to smoking, alcohol intolerance, or genetics, avoid using mouthwashes containing alcohol.

Look for an alcohol-free, antibacterial mouthwash instead of skipping the rinses altogether. More and more research links oral inflammation in the form of inflamed gums, teeth, and supporting bones to diabetes, atherosclerosis, heart disease, and stroke, as well as lung diseases like pneumonia and possibly even osteoporosis, arthritis, and Alzheimer's disease. Rinsing with mouthwash, brushing your teeth, and flossing can keep a lid on inflammation-causing organisms in your mouth.

No-cost tips for a germ-free toothbrush

It's true — toothbrushes can spread germs. But soaking yours in peroxide or buying a fancy sanitizer may not help. The American Dental Association (ADA) says there's no clinical evidence that soaks or special toothbrush sanitizers improve your health. Other suggestions, like putting your toothbrush through the dishwasher or in a microwave, can damage the bristles.

If you're set on buying a brush sanitizer, look for one approved by the Food and Drug Administration (FDA). This means the manufacturer has proven to the FDA that the product does what it claims.

Instead of spending your hard-earned cash, try these no-cost tips to keep your toothbrush germ-free.

- Rinse the bristles with water after brushing.

- Store the brush upright to air-dry, not in a closed container.

- Stand other people's toothbrushes so the heads and bristles don't touch to avoid transferring bacteria.

- Replace your brush every three to four months or when the bristles become noticeably frayed and worn, whichever comes first.

Medical alternatives

Play it safe during dental X-rays

Getting your teeth X-rayed only exposes you to a tiny bit of radiation, but it adds up. According to the National Academy of Sciences, there's no such thing as "safe" levels of radiation. With low doses, the cancer risk is small, but the exposure accumulates. The risk increases, over a lifetime.

Protect yourself during X-rays. Make sure your dentist or hygienist gives you a lead apron and a thyroid collar to wear, as the American Dental Association (ADA) recommends. Consider looking for a dentist who uses digital X-rays, also known as digital radiography. These can cut your radiation exposure by 70 to 80 percent compared to standard dental X-rays.

You may need bitewings and a panoramic X-ray when you see a new dentist for the first time. If you don't have cavities or a high risk for them, you should only need bitewings every two to three years after that. However, if you do tend to get cavities, you'll need them more often — every six to 18 months. On the other hand, if you have gum disease or another oral health problem, your dentist will decide how often you need X-rays. One more reason to take good care of your teeth.

Weigh the price of whitening

Whiter teeth may be all the rage, but the chemicals in at-home whiteners may do more harm than good because they soften your tooth enamel.

Most tooth enamel is naturally yellow-looking. Bleaching products use either hydrogen or carbamide peroxide to make your teeth appear whiter, but a recent study found that both strips and gel trays softened the hard, protective enamel coating your teeth.

They do work, however. A review of the research showed whitening strips with 5.5 to 6.5 percent hydrogen peroxide whitened better than gel trays containing 10 percent carbamide peroxide. These products weren't without side effects. People tended to complain of irritated gums and more sensitive teeth. The higher the hydrogen peroxide level, the more complaints.

Get other teeth and gum problems treated before you turn to whitening. The ADA says tooth decay, sensitive or cracked teeth, mouth infections, and gum problems need to be taken care of, first, because whitening may aggravate them. And remember, whitening only works on natural tooth enamel, not on crowns, veneers, bonding materials, or tooth-colored fillings.

Safer way to a brighter smile

Sensitive teeth need TLC, not strong chemicals. Bleaching products like whitening strips and gel trays aren't the only ways to brighten your teeth. Whitening toothpastes do the job more gently.

Some work by polishing teeth, through a chemical reaction, or by another non-bleaching method. Either way, they only remove surface stains, whereas bleaching products wipe out both surface and deep stains. No matter which product you choose to shine your pearly whites, look for the ADA Seal of Acceptance.

Ouch-free gum surgery

Surgery is a real pain, but sometimes it's the only way to treat receding gums. Luckily, a new technique could take the agony out of traditional gum-grafting procedures.

The normal method involves removing soft tissue from the palate, or roof, of your mouth and grafting it over the exposed roots of your teeth. The worst part may not be the gum graft itself but having tissue taken from the roof of your mouth, not to mention the stitches you end up with.

The new treatment solves that. Instead of grafting mouth tissue onto your gums, it uses high-tech patches made from collagen and treated with your own blood platelets. The surgeon then places these patches around your gums like a normal graft. It's less invasive and painful and has a shorter recovery time, although it's also more expensive and takes longer.

Defy your age with healthy skin

Save your skin from harm

Green tea can help you fight aging and, more importantly, beat the threat of skin cancer. Read on for vital information that can literally help you save your skin.

Fight wrinkles. Close to 90 percent of the visible signs of aging can be blamed on the ultraviolet (UV) rays hidden in sunlight. But when you drink green tea, you give your skin nutrients that can interfere with the wrinkle-making process. Here's how it works.

Youthful skin comes with its own anti-wrinkle and anti-sagging compounds. Collagen helps keep your skin firm while elastin helps your skin spring back after being stretched, pulled, or rubbed. Together, these compounds form a pattern that supports your skin the same way a wooden framework supports the walls of a house. Unfortunately, you may put your skin's framework in danger just by spending too much time in the sun.

The UV rays in sunlight encourage your body to overproduce free radical molecules, a problem that has been linked with skin aging and cancer. Those extra free radicals make your skin produce enzymes called metalloproteinases (MMPs), which break down collagen and elastin. Without enough collagen and elastin, your skin becomes less resilient and more prone to wrinkles and sags.

Fortunately, green tea contains powerful polyphenols that are also antioxidants. These polyphenol antioxidants act like a bomb squad against free radicals, neutralizing them before they can cause much damage. As a result, you get extra anti-wrinkle protection for your collagen, your elastin, and your skin. Studies suggest that both drinking green tea and applying green tea products to your skin may help. Just be sure to keep using sunscreen, too.

Repel cancer. Around 90 percent of all non-melanoma skin cancers are linked to sun exposure. Even worse, one out of every five Americans will develop skin cancer sometime in life — but you don't have to be one of them.

A study from Dartmouth Medical School found that people who drink two or more cups of black or green tea daily are less likely to get skin cancer. The researchers think this protection may come from the powerful antioxidants in tea. Tea polyphenols, like EGCG in green tea, may be particularly effective. What's more, animal studies suggest green tea and its polyphenols may protect you from cancer in four ways.

■ They may slash the number of MMPs sunlight can produce. Some of these MMPs help tumors grow.

■ They may protect your skin from free radical damage.

■ They decrease the levels of several substances that help tumor cells grow and develop their own blood vessels.

■ They boost compounds that cause cancer cells to commit suicide.

New ways to squash superbugs

Antibiotics normally get rid of infections, but those caused by antibiotic-resistant bacteria — or superbugs — can't be cured by most drugs. But surprising new research shows that green tea and Manuka honey may — like a can of Raid — help kill these superbugs dead.

- Out of 11 people hospitalized with antibiotic-resistant infections in the throat, eight got rid of their dangerous bacteria, often in 36 days or less, by drinking green tea daily while continuing their regular medical treatments.

- When Egyptian scientists pitted superbugs against antibiotics and green tea, 20 percent of the superbugs suddenly became receptive to antibiotics. The tea appeared to pump up the drugs' effectiveness, so taking your antibiotic with green tea might be a good idea.

- Infectious bacteria sometimes form colonies called biofilms that shield them from antibiotics. But recent research found that Manuka honey's bacteria-killing compounds can penetrate biofilms and help fight antibiotic-resistant bacteria.

Make wrinkles disappear naturally

Wrinkles, age spots, skin blemishes? Forget about buying expensive cosmetics and creams — you can keep your skin young and wrinkle-free using powerful, all natural nutrients that can also protect you from diseases such as cancer and heart disease. That's a double-duty benefit.

Reap the rewards of vitamin C. You can find plenty of exotic and expensive ingredients that promise perfect skin, but you don't want to miss the inexpensive vitamin that prevents the wrinkling caused by sun damage. As unlikely as it may sound, vitamin C can make a difference in your skin. A British study of over 4,000 women found that the ones who got less vitamin C were more likely to have wrinkles and dry skin. Apparently, vitamin C fights wrinkles in two ways.

- It helps your body make collagen, a compound that keeps your skin strong and flexible and helps repair skin when needed.

- It protects your skin cells from harmful free radicals and the skin damage they can cause.

But getting more vitamin C doesn't just help your skin. Studies have shown this powerful antioxidant can also protect you from cancer and heart disease. Consider these examples.

- People with the highest blood levels of vitamin C compared to the lowest were 42 percent less likely to have a stroke over 10 years, a study found.

- A review of nine large studies suggests that 700 mg of vitamin C daily may reduce your heart disease risk by up to 25 percent.

- Other research suggests that getting more vitamin C may lower your risk of at least five kinds of cancer.

To reap rewards like these, get as much vitamin C as possible from foods. Then talk to your doctor about whether supplements are right for you. Good sources of vitamin C include strawberries, sweet red peppers, papayas, cranberry juice cocktail, guavas, oranges, and pineapples.

Discover the power of linoleic acid. The same British study that uncovered the wrinkle-fighting power of vitamin C also detected another anti-aging nutrient — linoleic acid. You'll find this essential fatty acid in nuts, soybean oil, and green leafy vegetables.

The British scientists discovered that people who eat more linoleic acid may be less likely to develop dry, thinning skin. Linoleic acid turns into EPA and DHA in your body, the same omega-3 oils found in fatty fish. These oils may have the power to help protect your skin from the sun's damaging UV rays. And that may mean your skin stays young-looking longer.

Plump up your skin with water. When your skin doesn't get enough moisture, it not only gets brittle and dry, it becomes prone to wrinkles, too. Dermatologists say your skin depends on the water you drink for part of the moisture it needs. But many older adults do not get enough water.

Research shows that older adults are less likely to get thirsty when they're dehydrated. So you could be dehydrated and not even know it. In fact, that may help explain why hospital admissions for dehydration recently rose 40 percent over 10 years.

When you drink water regularly, your skin cells absorb that water and plump themselves up. This can help smooth away wrinkles caused by dehydration and rejuvenate your skin. It's like having a natural face lift. And you won't even need expensive creams or dangerous surgeries to do it.

Defend your skin with extra cancer fighters

Sunscreen may be the first step to keeping skin cancer away, but don't stop there. Add smart menu choices and high-powered nutrients to help make your skin even more resistant to skin cancer.

Save room for selenium. People with the highest blood levels of selenium may have less risk of skin cancer, a recent study found. One cause of this cancer is the dangerous free radical molecules generated in your skin when you're in the sun. Selenium is an antioxidant that neutralizes free radicals, making them harmless. This trace mineral may also rev up immune cells to help keep tumors from growing. Good sources of selenium include Brazil nuts, canned light tuna, cod, and light meat turkey.

Enjoy more carotenoids. Carotenoids may sound like creatures from outer space, but they're really nutritious pigments that give red, yellow, or orange color to foods like tomatoes, carrots, and corn. Carotenoids are also antioxidants that make themselves right at home in your skin after you eat them. So when too much sun exposure produces dangerous free radicals in your skin, carotenoid antioxidants can neutralize those free radicals on the spot.

Carotenoids may also increase the amount of blood passing through your skin. Because that blood flow delivers extra nutrients to your skin, carotenoids may improve your skin's ability to defend itself against dryness, roughness, and other effects of aging.

A tomato carotenoid called lycopene shows how well carotenoids can work. British researchers found that people who ate five tablespoons of tomato paste laced with olive oil every day for three months had 33 percent more protection against sunburn than people who just ate olive oil. They also had higher levels of a molecule that helps keep skin youthfully firm. You'll find lycopene in cooked tomato products like tomato paste, tomato soup, ketchup, and pasta sauce. You can also get other carotenoids from carrots and pomegranates.

Rediscover resveratrol. Grapes aren't just a cool juicy treat for hot weather. They're a leading source of a powerful compound called resveratrol, which may help prevent cancer in several ways.

- The equivalent of 45 grapes a day may protect important fats in your skin from sun damage, one study found.

- Resveratrol may trigger apoptosis, a process where cancer cells commit suicide.

- Animal studies suggest daily doses of resveratrol may help keep tumors from forming.

These are the kinds of protection that may help stop skin cancer before it starts. Get your resveratrol from grapes, peanuts, wine, and grape juice.

Go fish for omega-3 fatty acids. An Australian study found that people who eat more oily fish are less likely to get actinic keratosis, a precancerous skin condition. The researchers suspect that fish rich in omega-3s protect the skin against damage from inflammation, especially the kind caused by the sun. Less damage may mean less chance of precancerous spots. So enjoy up to 12 ounces of oily fish like herring, sardines, or trout every week.

Get to know niacin. Your skin's specialized immune system constantly works to protect you from cancer. But ultraviolet radiation from the sun may suppress that immune system, leaving you at higher danger of cancer. An Australian study recently found that 500 to 1,500 mg of vitamin B3 (niacin) every day may help fight the immune-blunting effects of UV radiation so your skin can stay safer. Even better, you can probably get that much vitamin B3 just by eating the right foods. Rich sources of vitamin B3 include fortified cereals, canned tuna, chicken, beef, and marinara sauce.

Other natural remedies

Natural protection against aging skin

Anti-aging creams and lotions may only be part of the secret to younger-looking skin. Natural supplements may help you get even better results by nourishing your skin from within.

Turn back the clock. Sweat and oil glands normally supply water and fats to help keep your skin smooth and soft. But, as you get older, your sweat and oil glands begin to waste away. As a result, your skin may become poorly hydrated, making it dry and scaly. But German scientists report that women who took a daily half-teaspoon of either borage oil or flaxseed oil for 12 weeks were rewarded with softer, better-hydrated skin.

Save your hide from sun damage. Getting older isn't the only thing that ages your skin. Sunlight can make things even worse. Exposure to the sun's ultraviolet (UV) rays can create too many free radical molecules in your skin. These trigger the breakdown of skin compounds like elastin and collagen, the connective tissues that keep your skin supple and wrinkle-free. That's like removing your skin's defense against wrinkles.

Fortunately, omega-3 fish oils may help. A British study found that people who took 10 grams — a little over two teaspoons — of omega-3 fish oil daily for six months became more resistant to erythema, a skin-reddening sign of sun damage. The researchers believe this means omega-3s can reduce the damaging effects of sunlight, thanks to their antioxidant powers. As a result, omega-3s can neutralize free radicals, prevent the destruction of your collagen, and help you avoid wrinkles.

Defend your skin. Lutein and zeaxanthin are nutritious pigments found in foods like leafy green vegetables and corn. Although they are more well-known for fighting macular degeneration and blindness, these nutrients may also help protect your skin from aging.

Exposure to the sun's UV rays can help dry out skin, leaving it without its protective layer of water and fats. But a study from Italy's University of Naples discovered that women who took 5 mg of lutein and zeaxanthin twice a day kept more protective fats in their skin than women who didn't. The supplements also improved skin hydration and elasticity, which may help keep your skin softer and more supple. Lutein and zeaxanthin may be well suited to help your skin for two reasons.

- They are antioxidants, which means they protect your skin against sun damage the same way fish oils do — by neutralizing free radicals.

- These nutrients go right into your skin, so they stand ready to defend it immediately at the first hint of trouble from sunlight.

Try a joint solution. You may have heard of glucosamine as an aid for joint pain and arthritis, but it may benefit skin, too. Because glucosamine encourages your body to make hyaluronic acid — a natural lubricator — it may also help decrease wrinkles and keep your skin better hydrated.

Talk to your doctor and pharmacist before trying supplements like these. Supplements may not be safe for people with certain health conditions and may interact with medications you already take. But if you get the green light, be sure to ask what brand of supplement your doctor or pharmacist recommends.

Battle psoriasis and win

Even severe psoriasis may get better if you choose the right supplement. A small study of people with severe erythrodermic psoriasis or arthropathic psoriasis found that those who took a daily supplement with their regular medical treatment saw more improvement in their condition than those who didn't. The supplement contained a combination of 50 mg of coenzyme Q10, 50 mg of vitamin E (alpha-tocopherol,) and 48 mcg of selenium. Talk to your doctor to find out whether this kind of supplement is right for you.

Healthful living

Kitchen essentials for younger-looking skin

The next time you're at a party, you may hear someone say, "I can't believe she's 70 ... she looks 50." Learn about using egg to make your face look younger along with seven other age-busting tips.

Egg. Some skin-care experts claim egg whites have skin-firming properties. So why not try an egg white mask and see for yourself? Just beat a single egg until frothy, and spread it on clean skin. As it dries, you may actually feel it tightening your skin. When dry, rinse with warm water.

Honey. Honey has been used by such famed beauties as Queen Cleopatra of ancient Egypt and Madame Du Barry of France — and perhaps with good reason. According to the National Honey Board, honey helps your skin attract and keep moisture, so it may be an ideal remedy for dryness. To give it a try, spread honey over your skin, and let it sit for 10-15 minutes before removing.

Honey may also ease two other skin problems. A small study suggests honey may help improve atopic dermatitis and common psoriasis. Study participants who got the best results applied a mixture of equal parts honey, beeswax, and olive oil directly on their skin.

Olive oil. In your pantry right now, you'll find an age-defying oil you can not only rub on your skin, but also take internally for added disease protection.

- Beauty experts recommend using olive oil in two ways. To exfoliate, combine six drops of olive oil with a tablespoon of sugar. Dampen your skin, massage the mixture in, and rinse with warm water. Also try using olive oil to wash and moisturize your face.

- Eat a Mediterranean diet rich in olive oil, and you may help protect yourself from heart disease and colon cancer. Unlike the standard American diet, the Mediterranean diet includes lots of fruits, veggies, whole grains, nuts, seeds, and beans. Sources of saturated fat, like red meats, dairy, and poultry, are often replaced by olive oil and other healthy fats. Olive oil helps improve high blood pressure, high triglycerides, and several other factors that raise your risk of heart disease. What's more, the phenols and monounsaturated fats in olive oil may help protect against cell changes and other processes that can lead to colon cancer.

Oatmeal. This grain can protect your skin from moisture loss, act as an exfoliant, and soothe irritated skin. That's exactly what you want in a dry-skin remedy, so try this one. Mix one-fourth cup of oatmeal with a half-cup of water, cook for two minutes, and let cool to warm. Stir in one-fourth cup of honey, apply to your face, let sit for 12 minutes, and rinse with cool water. The results may delight you.

Yogurt. Beauty experts say yogurt can exfoliate your skin and may even help your body make more collagen, thanks to its lactic acid. Make a yogurt night cream by squeezing half a lemon into a cup of yogurt. Stir and refrigerate. Each night, rub a dollop of this night cream on your face shortly before bedtime. Don't be surprised if you notice smoother, healthier skin in just a few weeks.

Cornmeal. If you need a gentler exfoliator, mix cornmeal with enough water to make a paste. Gently apply the mixture to your face. Let it dry and then lightly massage your skin. This helps remove dry, flaky skin, so the smoother skin beneath can shine through.

Lemon. Lemon juice may lighten age spots. Halve a lemon and squeeze its juice into a container. Use a cotton ball to apply the juice to your age spots, wait 20 minutes, and rinse. Do this three times a day. Stick with this routine, and your age spots may begin fading within a month.

Strawberry. Aim for more radiant skin with the best-smelling face mask ever. Mash strawberries and spread them across your face. Enjoy the heavenly scent for a few minutes and then rinse. You'll love the results.

5 sunscreen secrets you should know

Drive down your odds of sun damage, wrinkles, and skin cancer. With the right know-how, you can make sun protection stronger, simpler, and maybe even fun.

Your skin needs two kinds of protection. Ultraviolet (UV) A and UVB are the two types of rays that cause the sun's damaging effects. But the SPF number only tells how much protection you'll get from UVB rays. You also need protection against UVA rays, which are strong enough to penetrate window and windshield glass. These rays come in two skin-damaging forms, long wave and short wave. Check the ingredient list on your sunscreen label for oxybenzone to protect against the short-wave UVA rays. Then look for avobenzone, zinc oxide, titanium dioxide, or Mexoryl-SX to defend against long-wave UVA rays.

Sunblocks and sunscreens aren't the same. Sunblocks contain zinc oxide or titanium dioxide, compounds that reflect or "block" the sun's rays so they never reach your skin. Sunscreens, on the other hand, just filter and absorb UV rays, so they merely reduce the amount of sunlight that gets to your skin. Sunscreens also stop working after several hours in the sun, so plan to apply more every few hours for continuous age-fighting and cancer-fighting protection.

Sun-protecting make-up needs a boost. If you put on sunscreen or make-up with SPF, it can rub off within a few hours through sweat, snow, rain, or swimming. You should reapply your sunscreen during the day, even if you won't spend all your time in the sun.

Reapplying make-up, on the other hand, can be time-consuming, awkward, and possibly expensive. Fortunately, mineral make-up can help because it contains sunblocks like titanium dioxide or zinc oxide. If you can't reapply sunscreen, touch up your face with mineral powder throughout the day.

Lip gloss may raise your cancer risk. Lips can sunburn quickly, raising your odds of lip cancer. Make sure your lip balm or lipstick rates at least SPF 15 — preferably 30 — and reapply it regularly during the day. But don't wear shiny lip balms, lip glosses, or glossy lipsticks unless you wear SPF lip protection beneath. Glossy or shiny lip products may actually boost your risk of lip cancer.

Sunscreen-bug combos are a no-no. Avoid using combination sunscreen-insect repellent products. The insect repellent should only be put on once and very lightly, but sunscreen needs to be reapplied heavily every two hours.

Once you've protected yourself with sunscreen, don't stop there. Piling on extra sun protection not only keeps you cancer-free and young looking, it may also be fun.

- Take a tip from Hollywood stars and wear large sunglasses. You'll protect the delicate skin around your eyes.

- For a chic look, try long dresses or leggings that protect your legs from sunlight.

- Wear stylish broad-brimmed hats when outside. But before you wear a hat, hold it brim-side down in outdoor sunlight. If its shadow is flecked with light, pick a hat with a tighter weave.

And, of course, be sure to stay in the shade in the bright hours when your own shadow is short and UV light is at its worst.

Skin safety tips for CFLs

Sitting too close to a compact fluorescent bulb (CFL) may be risky for some people, new research suggests. Find out who is at risk and how easily you can protect yourself.

Research by the United Kingdom's Health Protection Agency found that some compact fluorescent light bulbs emit ultraviolet radiation — like the kind you get from sunlight. These amounts aren't enough to bother most people. But some people are particularly sensitive to light or ultraviolet radiation, especially those who have lupus, eczema, porphyria, chronic actinic dermatitis, or similar conditions. If you're one of those people, some CFL lights may be a source of harmful UV radiation for you.

But this danger only occurs if the light comes from an "open" spiral CFL and only if you stay within one foot of the bare bulb for an hour or more each day. You may be close enough if you use reading lamps, desk lamps, or similar task lighting.

Fortunately, protecting yourself is easy. Experts say you don't need to replace your bulbs if you always stay more than one foot away from the existing CFL bulb. If that's not practical, you can simply buy "encapsulated" or "double envelope" CFLs, the ones that look more like standard incandescent bulbs. The covers surrounding these bulbs help shelter you from ultraviolet radiation.

Meanwhile, don't worry about the long tube fluorescent lights that have been around for years. They're still safe to use in ceiling lights.

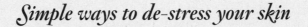

Simple ways to de-stress your skin

Stress can literally get under your skin. In fact, the American Academy of Dermatology says stress may prevent perfect skin in at least four ways.

- It makes your body release hormones and chemicals that promote inflammation and keep your skin from looking its best.

- It can worsen acne, psoriasis, rosacea, and other skin problems.

- It can help dehydrate your skin.

- During stressful moments, you may rub, scratch, or pull your skin, making your skin problems worse. During longer periods of stress, you may even forget to keep up the daily treatments and habits that can help your skin improve.

So start managing your stress. Read up on relaxation strategies. Listen to soothing music, try exercise like walking and gardening, or write in a diary. Not only will you feel better, you may start looking better, too.

Enjoy healthy, radiant skin for less

Expensive does not mean better when it comes to over-the-counter wrinkle creams, independent consumer testing found. What's more, even the best products tested made barely visible changes to wrinkles. So why not get healthier skin before you spend big bucks on wrinkle cream? Start with these inexpensive tips from the experts.

Beware the soap effect. Avoid using regular or deodorant soap to wash your face. As you age, your skin produces less of its natural oils and loses its ability to retain moisture. What's more, regular and deodorant soaps strip away oils and moisture, making your skin dry and rough. So wash your face with mild soap that contains moisturizers, or replace soap with a gentle cleanser.

Keep new wrinkles out. Skin naturally ages over time, but damage from sunlight has a much bigger impact than the passing years. That's why wrinkles usually occur in places where you've gotten the most sun exposure, such as your face. But one study of retirement home residents suggests it's never too late to begin protecting yourself from sun damage. You may benefit even now, so here's how to start.

- Stay out of the sun between 10 a.m. and 2 p.m., when UV radiation is at its worst.

- Wear moisturizer or foundation that contains sunscreen.

- Reapply sunscreen every few hours if you'll be outdoors awhile, even on overcast days.

See "5 sunscreen secrets you should know" on page 298 for more tips on effective sun protection.

Treat your face gently. After washing your face, don't rub it dry. Pat it instead and quickly apply moisturizer. Your moisturizer may not permanently erase wrinkles, but scientists say it may make wrinkles less noticeable.

Choose moisturizer wisely. According to experts, low-cost moisturizers can be just as effective as pricey department store buys. When choosing your moisturizer, remember these facts.

- Ingredients like glycerin and propylene glycol attract moisture to your skin while lanolin, silicone, petroleum jelly, or mineral oil keep moisture from escaping. Glycerin may be best for those with oily skin.

- Some moisturizers also have monolaurin, which may help your skin restore natural barriers against moisture loss.

- For added protection against skin aging, choose a moisturizer that contains sunscreen.

Exfoliate for better skin. When you're 20, your skin automatically sheds older skin cells and replaces them with younger ones, so you get a youthful new topcoat every month. But your skin-shedding ability naturally declines as you age, so you need to exfoliate to get rid of dead skin cells.

You can either buy an exfoliating product or find a good exfoliator in another product like a moisturizer. The best exfoliators are alpha hydroxy acids (AHAs) and beta hydroxy acids (BHAs.) Types of AHAs include lactic acids from milk, malic acid from apples, citric acid from oranges or lemons, and tartaric acid from grapes. But the most common AHA is glycolic acid from sugar cane. Look for a product with 8 to 10 percent AHAs. If the label doesn't give you a percentage, check the ingredient list. The AHA should be one of the first few ingredients.

Another plus is that AHAs may stimulate the production of collagen and elastin, which help keep your skin supple and resilient. That gives you an extra defense against wrinkles.

While AHAs are best for dry skin, BHAs like salicylic acid are better for oily skin and may be less irritating. BHAs work best at a concentration of 1 to 2 percent. Be aware that both acids may irritate your skin and make it more sensitive to the sun. So if you use BHAs or AHAs, wear sunscreen all day, every day.

Savvy secrets for wrinkle-cream buyers

Over-the-counter (OTC) wrinkle creams may not make you look 17 again, but they can offer some help. Just be sure to read ingredient lists, and choose carefully.

Many studies have confirmed the benefits of retinol, so look for this ingredient on wrinkle-cream labels. Unfortunately, since OTC wrinkle creams are unregulated, you may have a tough time telling whether a product has enough retinol to make a difference. Call the product maker for more information, or talk to your dermatologist. A concentration of 0.2 is enough, but it will make you more sensitive to sunlight and may irritate your skin.

Antioxidant ingredients are also promising. Vitamin C may be the best one because it has the most studies backing its effectiveness. Keep an eye out for it when you're checking labels.

Other compounds — like green tea, lutein, zeaxanthin, alpha-lipoic acid, and oligomeric proanthocyanidins — have shown promise in early studies, so stay tuned to see if they work.

Smart ways to battle 'superbugs'

Dangerous antibiotic-resistant infections don't just happen to people in hospitals anymore. Now 12 percent of those illnesses occur in people who haven't been anywhere near a hospital. What's more, 59 percent of the skin infections diagnosed in city emergency rooms were antibiotic-resistant, one study reports. But don't raise the white flag yet. These infections often are curable, and you can still protect yourself.

Know your enemy. Many perfectly healthy people carry bacteria called *Staphylococcus aureus*, or staph, in their noses or on their skin. Staph is one of the most common sources of skin infections in the United States. But all staph aren't created equal — some strains of staph are resistant to antibiotics. These are called methicillin-resistant *Staphylococcus aureus* (MRSA). That means certain antibiotics like penicillin or amoxicillin can't kill these bacteria.

When staph infections occur in people who haven't been in a hospital, they're called community associated (CA). They can be caused by both regular staph and MRSA. In healthy people, CA infections often show up as pimples or boils that may be red and swollen, and may even have pus or other drainage.

Doctors can treat most staph and MRSA infections. The death rate for CA-MRSA infections is only one out of every 200,000 people or, for those over age 65, two out of every 100,000 people. But it pays to play it safe.

Look for ways to avoid MRSA. Simple tips like these can help keep CA-MRSA away.

■ Wash your hands often. Direct skin-to-skin contact with any contaminated person can infect you. Keep wounds, cuts, or abrasions covered with a clean, dry bandage, and practice proper wound treatment and care until the area has healed.

■ Don't share. Because MRSA can live on objects like doctor's clothing and dish towels, you can get infected by touching these items. So don't share soap, towels, razors, or other things that have come into contact with another person's skin. Again, wash your hands, or use alcohol-based hand sanitizer, especially when visiting or leaving any doctor's office, clinic, or hospital.

■ Practice safe sneezing. Studies suggest that sneezing may spread MRSA through the air. If you don't have a tissue, sneeze into the crook of your arm, and encourage others to do the same.

Protect your pets and yourself. A recent study found you can get MRSA from pets — and give it to them, too. Take these precautions if you have animals.

■ Make sure your pets get the recommended veterinary care, including shots and treatments to control parasites.

■ Keep your pets clean, and wash your hands after touching them or cleaning up after them.

■ When choosing a pet, stick with the traditional kinds like dogs or cats. Avoid exotic pets and wild animals who may be more likely to carry MRSA or other contagious diseases.

■ Avoid letting pets lick you, and don't kiss them.

■ Keep any open wounds on you or your pet covered when you're together.

If you must be treated for MRSA, ask your vet whether your pet needs treatment, too.

Fend off health dangers of psoriasis

Having psoriasis may put you at higher risk of developing diabetes or high blood pressure. Scientists aren't sure how these health problems are connected, but inflammation is a prime suspect because it probably plays a role in all three conditions. Plans to study this possible inflammation link are already in the works, so stay tuned.

Meanwhile, if you have psoriasis, take special precautions with your health. Talk to your doctor about your risk of diabetes and high blood pressure, and ask what steps you can take to prevent them.

Pick your soap carefully

Skip the antibacterial soap, especially those that contain triclosan. Unlike soap or alcohol-based cleaners, triclosan doesn't wipe out all the bacteria in sight. Instead, some studies say it wipes out most of the bacteria, leaving the triclosan-resistant bacteria free to take over. Some studies even suggest the bacteria that resist triclosan may be more likely to resist antibiotics, too.

Some studies have found that "antibacterial" hand soaps and cleaners are no better than regular cleaners at preventing infections like colds and flu simply because many infections are caused by viruses rather than bacteria. In a study of health care workers whose hands were deliberately coated with flu virus, researchers found two methods of removal to be the most effective.

■ Wash hands with soap and water. Work the soap into your hands for at least 15 seconds, and rinse thoroughly.

- Use an alcohol-based hand sanitizer with at least 60 percent alcohol. Make sure you use enough sanitizer that your hands take at least 20 seconds to dry. It takes the alcohol that long to kill the bacteria.

If someone in your household is pregnant or has a compromised immune system, you should check with their doctor first before making any changes to the cleaners you use.

Double your defense against shingles

About one out of three adults in the United States will get shingles, a painful skin condition. And more than a third of those will develop serious complications like postherpetic neuralgia (PHN) — severe pain that may last months or years. A vaccine to combat the disease only prevents 50 percent of shingles cases and 67 percent of PHN cases. But the good news is you can double your defense by combining the vaccine with a non-drug solution that helps strengthen your immune system.

Tai chi is the secret weapon. A recent study found that this gentle martial art may turbocharge your immunity against shingles. In the study, two groups of older adults took classes three times a week for four months. One group took tai chi classes while the other took health education classes. Afterward, both groups were tested to gauge their immunity against shingles.

The tai chi group's resistance to shingles improved so much that it nearly matched the immunity they'd have gotten from taking the vaccine. And when the tai chi group actually received the shingles vaccine, their immunity improved to levels normally seen in middle-aged adults — even though many study participants were past middle age.

In the end, the tai chi group had twice as much immunity to shingles as the health education group. The tai chi group also reaped other benefits such as better mental health and the ability to do everyday tasks more easily.

Scent-sational way to reverse hair loss

Start winning the battle against hair loss. Here is what you need to know.

Pinpoint the "mane" problem. It pays to know which kind of hair loss you have. Some people develop temporary hair loss from causes like medication, a recent illness, or hair bleaching. Others, including women, inherit "male pattern" baldness (androgenetica alopecia) from their parents or other relatives. But if you lose small, round patches of hair on your scalp, face, or chest, you may have aleopecia areata, an immune disorder that causes your immune system to attack your hair follicles.

To find out which kind of hair loss you have, talk to your doctor. If she says you have alopecia areata, an unusual but delightful remedy may help.

Stimulate hair growth. The scents of lavender, rosemary, thyme, and cedar could provide a spa-style solution to your hair loss. In a Scottish study, two groups of people with alopecia areata were asked to massage a mix of aromatherapy oils into their scalps for at least two minutes every night. One group used carrier oils like grapeseed and jojoba, while the other group used a mixture of essential oils.

The "magic" mixture included 2 drops of thyme oil (*Thyme vulgaris*), 3 drops of lavender oil (*Lavandula augustifolia*), 3 drops of rosemary oil (*Rosmarinus officinalis*), 2 drops of cedarwood oil

(*Cedrus atlantica*), roughly 4 1/4 teaspoons of grapeseed oil, and nearly 3/4 teaspoon of jojoba oil.

After seven months, three times as many members of the essential oil group showed improvement as those in the other group. The researchers even had before and after pictures to prove it. And according to the pictures, one study participant who was nearly bald regained almost all of his hair. So try this hair root stimulator, and get out your comb.

Get your doctor's OK. If you'd like to try this treatment, check with your doctor or dermatologist first. Plant oils may cause side effects or allergic reactions in some people, particularly those who take medication or have other medical conditions. If your doctor gives you the green light, be sure to include the grapeseed and jojoba carrier oils. These help protect you from getting unsafe amounts of the essential oils in the mixture.

Medical alternatives

---

8 ways to kiss wrinkles good-bye

Sagging skin got your spirit dragging? A new nonsurgical face lift may be just what the doctor ordered. From chemical peels to laser resurfacing, new technology allows you to have younger-looking skin.

"I had the procedure done two-and-a-half weeks ago and I love it," said 48-year old Margaret after her nonsurgical face lift. "My skin is smooth. The brown spots on my face are gone. It makes me feel much younger. It just feels good to look in the mirror."

If you're interested in a nonsurgical face lift, here are a few of the options you should know about.

Procedure	What it is	Pros	Cons	Follow-up
Botox injection $391	A tiny amount of purified botulism toxin is injected into the muscles that cause wrinkles in order to paralyze them.	Good for frown lines, forehead lines, lines between the lips and nose, and crow's feet. Can be done in less than an hour and requires no recovery period.	May cause temporary discomfort, muscle weakness, or bruising. Risk of bruising, numbness, or swelling. May make frowning or squinting more difficult.	May need repeat treatments every three to six months.
Chemical peel $815	Uses various kinds of chemicals to strip off the top layer of skin so newer skin can grow back. Peel may be light (superficial), medium, or deep.	Good for facial wrinkles, age spots, fine lines, or large pores.	Can cause temporary throbbing, swelling, redness, flaking, and sun sensitivity. Redness and peeling may last several days or weeks. May also cause cold sores, infection, scarring, skin allergies, and permanent discoloration in some people.	A medium peel lasts up to two years. May need to be repeated annually.
Ablative laser skin resurfacing $2,128	Uses laser light to remove some skin and tighten the remaining skin. May also stimulate collagen production.	Good for wrinkles around the mouth and eyes.	Temporary throbbing pain after surgery that may require pain medication. Side effects may also include burns, skin lightening, and bruising. May have a recovery period of up to two weeks. Skin redness may last several months.	May last 10 years but may require more than one treatment to get final results.

Procedure	What it is	Pros	Cons	Follow-up
Nonablative laser skin resurfacing (Fractional) $1,359	New fractionated lasers remove thousands of closely spaced microscopic columns of skin, leaving surrounding skin untouched. Stimulates production of collagen.	Good for wrinkles, scars, sun damage, and more. Each treatment takes one hour or less.	May experience pain, swelling, redness and flaking but can cover with cosmetics immediately. Recovery period may last up to five days.	May require three to six treatments. Results vary and may last from one to five years.
Microderm-abrasion $200	Uses microscopic particles or a diamond-tipped wand to "sand off" or remove some of the topmost layer of skin so new skin will grow.	Good for fine lines, age spots, and crow's feet. Can be done quickly and requires no recovery period.	Temporary redness. Risk of swelling and sensitivity.	Requires five or six sessions spaced two weeks apart. May last about three years.

Procedure	What it is	Pros	Cons	Follow-up
Collagen injection $452 (animal) $467 (human)	Injection of collagen from cows, pigs, or humans reduces facial wrinkles caused by loss of fat or collagen.	Good for scars and wrinkles. Takes less than an hour and has no recovery time.	Risk of allergic reaction to bovine collagen. May require advance allergy testing.	Lasts three to six months depending on type chosen.
Hyaluronic injection $578	Injection of hyaluronic acid reduces facial wrinkles caused by loss of fat or collagen.	Good for scars and wrinkles. Takes less than an hour and has no recovery time.	More likely to cause swelling, redness, bruising, and pain than collagen.	Lasts six to 12 months.
Artefill injectable implant $2,100	Injection of polymethyl-methacrylate (PMMA) with bovine collagen that smoothes away wrinkles.	Used for forehead wrinkles, wrinkles between the lip and nose, and for scars. Less painful than hyaluronic injections.	Risk of swelling, redness, and lumpiness. May require allergy testing in advance.	Lasts at least five years and is often permanent.

FDA issues Botox warning

Botox can cause symptoms like difficulty breathing or severe difficulty with swallowing in some people, warns the Food and Drug Administration (FDA). Here's what you need to know.

These side effects are most likely to occur in people who use Botox as a treatment for excessive neck muscle contractions or severe muscle tightness. The FDA is not sure whether these side effects are possible with other uses of Botox, such as treatment of frown lines between the eyebrows, crossed eyes, severe underarm sweating, and abnormal eyelid twitches.

But if you have used Botox within the last few weeks and experience any of the following symptoms, seek medical help immediately: unexpected muscle weakness, trouble talking or saying words clearly, blurred vision, drooping eyelids, double vision, loss of bladder control, trouble breathing, or trouble swallowing.

Cut your shingles risk in half

That case of chickenpox you had as a child can turn into something far more dangerous and painful as you age — shingles. Fortunately, a new vaccine may help you avoid the agonizing pain it causes and the scary complications that may follow.

Shingles is caused by the same virus that gives you chickenpox. After your immune system trounces the chickenpox, the virus can stay dormant in your nerves for decades. But as you grow older, your immunity to the virus may weaken, and you can develop a painful, band-shaped rash of blisters. This rash can be so sensitive that a breeze or the weight of clothing can be excruciating. But eventually the blisters drain and scab over and most people get better. However, others develop complications like postherpetic neuralgia (PHN) — intense pain that may linger for months or years. Some may even develop vision or hearing problems.

Protect yourself. Antivirals can help if you get treatment soon enough, but it's better to avoid shingles in the first place. That's where the new vaccine comes in.

As you age, your odds of getting shingles go up. So the Centers for Disease Control and Prevention (CDC) recommends you get the Zostavax vaccine if you're age 60 or older — even if you've already had shingles and recovered. Research suggests that getting this shot reduces your risk of shingles by 50 percent and lessens the severity of shingles if you get it. Even better, the vaccine slashes your odds of PHN by 67 percent. While the vaccine may become less effective at preventing shingles as you age, it continues to prevent PHN just as well after age 70 as it does during your 60s.

Check it out. The Zostavax vaccine is relatively new so remember these tips.

- Call your insurance provider first to find out how much of the cost of the shot is covered. The total fee may range from $165 to $300. The cost of a case of shingles, however, can be significantly higher.

- Check with your doctor's office to see if it offers the vaccine. If not, try a walk-in clinic at your local drugstore.

■ You aren't likely to get shingles from the vaccine, but some people may get side effects like pain, swelling, or tenderness in the spot where they get the shot. A few may even experience itching or a headache.

Be careful. This vaccine isn't for everyone. For example, you shouldn't get vaccinated if you're currently taking immune-suppressing drugs, if you've ever had a severe allergic reaction to neomycin or gelatin, or if you have ever had an immune-deficiency condition like leukemia. Also, don't get vaccinated if you currently have shingles or PHN. Instead, let your doctor know you have shingles right away so he can treat you with anti-viral medication.

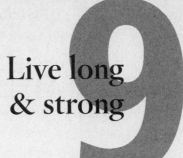

Live long
& strong

Surprising solution for chronic pain

Getting older doesn't mean you have to live with aches and pains.
You also don't have to depend on high doses of pain pills for relief.
Easing the discomfort can be as easy as boosting your intake of
vitamin D.

Low levels, high risk. A recent University of Delaware study of
older people in the Chianti region of Italy found that older women
who aren't getting enough vitamin D may be at higher risk for back
pain. Other studies have found similar links.

A review of 22 clinical studies found that people with chronic body
aches and back pain usually had low levels of vitamin D. Luckily,
once they began getting enough, those aches and pains often diminished or even disappeared. For example, after taking vitamin D
supplements for three months, 95 percent of people with chronic
back pain in one study reported improvement.

Besides back pain, vitamin D may also help with bone and joint pain, osteoarthritis, rheumatoid arthritis, fibromyalgia, diabetic neuropathy, chronic fatigue syndrome, and seasonal affective disorder, or SAD.

How it helps. Your body needs vitamin D to absorb calcium. When you don't get enough, it takes calcium from your bones, weakening them and possibly leading to fractures. The outer layer of bones can also become soft and spongy. This spongy layer may expand and press against sensitive tissues covering your bones, a painful condition called osteomalacia. Raising your intake of vitamin D can improve calcium absorption and keep your bones and muscles strong.

Don't think of vitamin D as a miracle cure. Because vitamin D tackles the underlying cause of pain rather than the pain itself, it may take weeks or months before you notice any improvement. While vitamin D may not entirely replace your pain medication, it may ease your pain and lessen the need for drugs.

Super sources. Your skin produces vitamin D when it's exposed to sunlight. You can also find vitamin D in some food sources. Fatty fish like salmon, herring, mackerel, sardines, and tuna are your best bets. Fortified foods, such as milk, cheese, and cereal, also provide vitamin D. You can even get a small amount from egg yolks.

But to get enough vitamin D, you likely need supplements. Experts recommend taking at least 1,000 international units (IU) of vitamin D a day if you're healthy and up to 2,000 IU if you have pain. Do not take more than that without a doctor's supervision. Vitamin D supplements are cheap and readily available. Look for vitamin D-3, the form naturally produced by your skin.

For more information about vitamin D, please see "Beat disease with the sunshine vitamin" on page 82 in *Cardio health: fit for life*.

Fight muscle loss with chocolate milk

You may get weaker as you get older, but your refrigerator contains some strong weapons to help you fight back.

Sarcopenia, the loss of muscle mass and function that comes with aging, hampers your mobility, makes you weak, and increases your risk of falls. Luckily, you can partially reverse sarcopenia with exercise, particularly strength training. If you're trying to build up your muscle strength, you can start by adding these tasty and helpful foods to your strength-building program.

Milk. Can a glass of sweet milk slow the aging process? Yes, if you drink it immediately after a workout. The research sounds unbelievable until you read how it works in your body.

A small study found that older women benefited from sweetened milk immediately after a strength training session. Drinking this combination of carbohydrates and protein helped increase their skeletal muscle, leading researchers to speculate that it could be a good way to counteract muscle loss with aging.

In an earlier study of male cyclists, chocolate milk worked better than commercial sports drinks, helping them recover and cycle longer in their next workout. A recent Canadian review pointed out that low-fat milk is as effective as sports drinks for recovery after strength and endurance training. Drinking milk after exercising will help your muscles increase in size and strength, while promoting the loss of body fat.

Cherries. Drinking cherry juice before and after workouts may lessen muscle pain and damage, according to a small University of Vermont study. College students who drank 12 ounces of tart cherry juice twice a day for eight days had significantly less pain and strength loss after performing arm exercises than those who drank a placebo beverage. Strength loss was 22 percent in the placebo group, but only 4 percent for the cherry juice drinkers. The antioxidant and anti-inflammatory powers of cherries likely provided the benefits. Twelve fluid ounces of cherry juice is equivalent to 50 to 60 tart cherries.

Fruits and veggies. One recent study found that higher intakes of foods rich in potassium, like fruits and vegetables, not only keeps your blood pressure in check but can help preserve muscle strength and prevent disability as you age. Eating too much protein and cereal grains makes your blood too acidic, causing muscle tissue to waste away. On the other hand, the potassium in fruits and vegetables makes your blood more alkaline and increases your lean muscle mass.

Of course, getting more potassium — and less sodium — into your diet is also a great way to prevent or lower high blood pressure and reduce your risk of strokes.

In addition to eating more fruits and vegetables, you should also drink less soda. Excessive cola consumption can lead to hypokalemia, a condition in which potassium levels fall and vital muscle function suffers. Symptoms range from mild weakness to paralysis. Luckily, if you stop drinking cola and take supplemental potassium, it's easy to recover. The glucose, fructose, and caffeine in colas each contribute to the problem.

Lean meat. You need fewer calories as you age — but you still need just as much protein. Unfortunately, many older people don't get enough. When that happens, your body must raid your muscles for the amino acids it needs to keep your organs working. Eventually, that lost muscle leads to weakness.

Cost, difficulty chewing, and a decline in appetite may explain why older people don't eat enough protein. Make an effort to boost your protein intake. It could help slow the deterioration of your muscles. One study found that eating more protein even reduces wrist fractures because it's good for bone health.

Experts suggest aiming for 1 gram of protein per kilogram of body weight, which is roughly equal to half your weight in pounds, each day. That means if you weigh 160 pounds you should eat 80 grams of protein every day. Good sources include beef, pork, chicken, fish, eggs, dairy, and nuts.

You can also get protein from protein powders, which claim to build muscle. Most have 100 to 150 calories per serving and deliver 30 to 60 percent of the protein you need each day. Just add a scoop to your yogurt or smoothie. One good option is whey protein. Its high concentration of the amino acid leucine may help older people maintain muscle mass. Studies show it helps minimize sarcopenia. It can also help you maintain a healthy weight by controlling your appetite.

Nutrients that help prevent falls

Over half the falls among older people result in an injury. While most of these injuries aren't life-threatening, no one wants to risk a fracture — or worse. You can protect yourself from falls just by eating foods rich in these nutritional powerhouses.

Vitamin D. Studies show the sunshine vitamin has a positive effect on muscle strength and balance. It also helps maintain bone density.

One three-year study found that taking vitamin D and calcium reduced the risk of falls in older women by 46 percent. Among less-active women, it was even more helpful, slashing fall risk by 65 percent. Vitamin D deficiency has been linked to muscle weakness, and older people may lose some vitamin D receptors in their muscles with age.

A Dutch study found that older people with a vitamin D deficiency were more likely to fall multiple times during a 12-month period than those getting an adequate amount of vitamin D. Those low on vitamin D were 78 percent more likely to fall twice, and their risk of falling three or more times more than doubled.

In an Australian study, vitamin D supplements helped women with a history of falling and low blood levels of vitamin D. It reduced the risk of having at least one fall by 19 percent. It also helped more in the winter, when blood levels of vitamin D are lower because of decreased exposure to the sun.

Spending 10 to 15 minutes in the sun a few times a week may help boost your vitamin D levels. You can also get vitamin D from liver, egg yolks, and oily fish like salmon, mackerel, tuna, and sardines. Foods fortified with vitamin D include milk, orange juice, and breakfast cereals. Multivitamins often contain vitamin D, and you can also take supplements.

Vitamin E. A recent study in Tuscany, Italy, determined that low levels of vitamin E were associated with physical decline in older people. Tasks to measure physical decline included walking speed, repeated chair rises, and standing balance. Those low in vitamin E were 62 percent more likely to show signs of physical decline during the three-year follow-up.

Because vitamin E acts as an antioxidant, low levels could mean increased oxidative stress, leading to muscle or DNA damage. Vitamin E deficiency has also been linked to atherosclerosis and other cardiovascular diseases, as well as brain disorders.

Some health experts suggest aiming for 15 to 30 milligrams (mg) of vitamin E a day. That's easy to get through food sources, such as almonds, tomato sauce, and sunflower seeds. Wheat germ, dark leafy greens, vegetable oils, and other nuts and seeds also provide vitamin E.

Carotenoids. These pigments in food range from light yellow to reddish orange. Like beta carotene, the most common carotenoid, these phytochemicals act as antioxidants. Other carotenoids include lycopene, lutein, and zeaxanthin.

A recent Italian study found that high blood concentrations of carotenoids may help you stay steady on your feet. Those with the highest levels were about half as likely to have trouble walking. They also had a less-steep decline in walking speed during a six-year follow-up.

You can get carotenoids from colorful fruits and vegetables, such as apricots, broccoli, cantaloupe, carrots, pumpkin, spinach, sweet potatoes, and tomatoes.

Stay hydrated to stay steady

The right foods can keep you on solid footing — but don't forget about liquids. Drinking plenty of water is also key to maintaining your balance.

Dehydration can cause dizziness and potentially serious falls. It can also lead to constipation, confusion, and fatigue. Unfortunately, many older people do not drink enough water. As you get older, your body becomes less able to sense dehydration and signal your brain that you're thirsty.

Drinking more water can help. One nursing home in England reported dramatic results when it encouraged its residents to drink 10 glasses of water a day. There were half as many falls and fewer calls for doctors. The nursing home also saw a decrease in laxative use and urinary infections, improvement in sleep quality, and less agitation among residents with dementia.

How much water do you need? One common guideline is eight 8-ounce glasses of water a day. But some experts have called that recommendation into question. That's because you get much of the water you need from food and other beverages. Fruits and vegetables, like watermelon and tomatoes, provide a lot of water. So do milk, juice, and even caffeinated beverages like coffee, tea, and soda.

There's also a danger of drinking too much water. This can dilute your electrolytes, a condition called water intoxication. Severe cases may be life threatening. In at least one case, a 45-year-old woman developed water intoxication by drinking large quantities of water to suppress her appetite. Even during heavy exertion in high heat, the U.S. Army has warned its members against drinking more than six 8-ounce glasses of water in an hour or more than 48 8-ounce glasses in 12 hours.

But most people need to worry more about drinking enough water rather than drinking too much. You especially need to boost your water intake in hot and humid weather, when you exercise, and during illness. Under normal circumstances, try drinking a glass of water with each meal and between each meal. Plus, of course, when you're thirsty.

Foil fatigue with quercetin

You know you should exercise regularly, but it's tough to stay motivated, especially when you get tired quickly. Fortunately, quercetin can help. This natural polyphenolic flavonoid, found in onions, apples, grapes, and berries, gives a boost to your muscles and your brain.

Quercetin works by increasing the number of mitochondria — the tiny powerhouses within cells that burn fuel — in your muscles and brain. This leads to greater endurance and a greater willingness and motivation to exercise. In one study, mice voluntarily ran faster and about 35 percent farther on a wheel after six days of quercetin treatment.

Mitochondria and exercise are closely linked. When your mitochondria don't work properly, it lowers your body's tolerance for exercise — and lack of exercise is a risk factor for developing diseases like diabetes, cancer, and heart disease. Exercising doubles the number and performance of mitochondria in muscle. But exercise programs can be hard to start and maintain.

That's where quercetin comes in. By boosting mitochondria, quercetin can help you overcome two big deterrents to exercise — tiring quickly and lack of motivation. That's because mitochondria have a big impact on physical endurance. Boosting mitochondrial function helps cells suck up more oxygen, delaying fatigue. In one human study, a combination of quercetin, caffeine, and other antioxidants taken for six weeks improved bicycle exercise endurance. Mitochondria also play a role in motivation and mood, including vigor, fatigue, anxiety, and depression.

Besides food sources, quercetin is found in products such as FRS energy drinks, mixes, and chews and RealFX Q-Plus Chews.

6 nutritional tips for better sleep

Trouble sleeping? Sleeping pills are not the answer. Try a few simple changes to your diet instead. Put the right foods on your plate, and spend more quality time with your head on the pillow.

Sleeping problems get worse with age. Instead of sleeping like a baby, you may have trouble falling asleep or staying asleep. Changes in your body clock contribute to insomnia, as do illnesses and the medications used to treat them. Insomnia can increase your risk for depression, memory problems, daytime sleepiness, and nighttime falls. Good sleep hygiene can help. So can the following dietary tips.

Choose cherries. Rather than rely on sleeping pills, try this fruit instead. Loaded with a natural hormone that helps "shut off" your wakeful brain, cherries could be the perfect bedtime snack. Studies show that melatonin improves the quality of sleep and boosts blood levels of melatonin in older people with insomnia. It also shortens the time needed to fall asleep. Cherries are a good source of melatonin, which is readily absorbed by your body. A handful of cherries a day should provide all the melatonin you need. You can also buy melatonin supplements. Research suggests the best dosage is 0.3 milligrams (mg) a day.

Make room for magnesium. Research shows high magnesium levels may help people fall asleep faster and sleep more soundly. Good sources of magnesium include nuts, legumes, whole grains, dark leafy greens, and seafood.

Count on carbohydrates. An Australian study found that starchy carbohydrates eaten four hours before bedtime help people fall asleep faster. That's because these carbohydrates may boost levels of tryptophan and serotonin, two brain chemicals involved in sleep. Although the study used jasmine rice, you can try other types of carbohydrates that rank high on the Glycemic Index, which measures how quickly foods raise your blood sugar. Good options include mashed potatoes, bagels, saltine or Graham crackers, jelly beans, French bread, pretzels, and rice cakes.

Trim the fat. Several studies show that fatty foods give you a fat chance for a good night's sleep. A study of Chinese men and women found that people who slept less than seven hours a night ate more fat than those who slept seven to nine hours a night. An Israeli study of mice found that a high-fat diet affects the body clock, disrupting the sleep cycle. Brazilian researchers also found that total fat intake and fat intake at dinner negatively affect sleep patterns.

Lay off late-night snacks. Eating high-calorie late-night snacks can lead to awakenings during sleep, according to a Brazilian study. In fact, eating too many calories during the day may lead to interruptions in your sleep.

Eliminate energy drinks. If you're tired after a fitful night's sleep, don't turn to energy drinks for an extra burst of energy. These products contain lots of caffeine — up to 141 mg per serving, more than an 8-ounce cup of coffee — and can lead to elevated blood pressure and heart rate. They're also loaded with sugar, sodium, and calories — often 200 or more per serving. Too much caffeine can cause increased heart rate, restlessness, anxiety, and nausea, as well as sleep deprivation. Worse, you may not know how much caffeine you're getting because the label doesn't always show this information.

Breathe easier with lung friendly foods

Lung disease takes your breath away — literally. When you have chronic obstructive pulmonary disease (COPD), you experience wheezing, coughing, and shortness of breath. Even eating may be too tiring. But it's important to eat a healthy diet. The right foods can help you cope with this condition — or even prevent it in the first place.

COPD refers to two lung conditions, emphysema and chronic bronchitis, which frequently go hand-in-hand. In both conditions, airflow is blocked, impairing your breathing. Smoking is the main cause of COPD, the fourth-leading cause of death in the United States. Other risk factors include exposure to air pollution, second-hand smoke, and occupational dusts and chemicals. Heredity and a history of childhood respiratory infections can also play a role.

Half of all people with COPD say their condition limits their ability to work. It also takes its toll on household chores, sleeping, and social and family activities. People who have COPD often become thin because eating becomes a chore, and the struggle of breathing burns more calories than it does in healthy people.

Standard treatment options include quitting smoking, medication, supplemental oxygen, and surgery. But your diet can also make a difference.

You are what you eat. Researchers found a stark difference between what they deemed a "prudent pattern" of eating and a typical Western pattern. The prudent pattern is rich in fruits, vegetables, fish, and whole grain products, while the Western pattern is rich in refined grains, cured and red meats, desserts, and French fries.

In one study, men who followed the prudent pattern cut their risk of COPD in half, while those who ate the Western diet more than quadrupled their risk. A separate study of women found similar results. Women who stuck to the prudent pattern cut their risk by

25 percent, and those who followed the Western diet boosted their risk by 31 percent. Here are some other things to consider.

- Tomato juice prevented emphysema from developing in mice exposed to cigarette smoke. The antioxidant power of lycopene, the carotenoid that gives tomatoes their red color, could get the credit, but other parts of the tomato may play a role, too.

- The higher the level of vitamin D in your blood, the better your lungs function. You can get vitamin D from foods like fatty fish, liver, egg yolks, and fortified milk and cereal.

- Eat more fiber for better lung function and reduced risk of COPD. Cereal and fruit fiber were most helpful in one study. Researchers suspect the anti-inflammatory and antioxidant properties of fiber may help.

A few studies show the danger of cured meats, such as bacon, sausage, hot dogs, and luncheon meats. Eating these foods frequently can reduce your lung function and boost your risk of COPD. One study found that those who ate the most cured meats were more than twice as likely to develop COPD as those who ate the least. For each single increase in cured meat servings a month, the risk of COPD goes up 2 percent, according to another study. Nitrites in cured meats are likely to blame, because they generate free radicals that may cause lung damage.

Smart eating strategies. If you already have COPD, try these tips to make eating easier and healthier.

- Eat five or six small meals a day instead of three large ones. Your stomach won't fill up as much, giving your lungs more room to expand.

- Drink plenty of fluids to avoid dehydration. Drink beverages at the end of your meal so you don't fill up too soon.

- Add a liquid protein supplement to your diet to prevent weight loss.

- Eat and chew slowly. Avoid foods that are difficult to chew.

- Avoid foods that cause gas or bloating.

- Skimp on salt. Too much can cause you to retain fluids, which may interfere with breathing.

- Don't waste energy eating foods with little nutritional value, such as chips, candy, or soft drinks.

- Choose foods that are easy to prepare, so you don't spend all your energy cooking instead of eating.

- Enjoy high-calorie snacks if you need to put on weight. Options include ice cream, cookies, pudding, cheese, crackers with peanut butter, bagels with cream cheese, fruits and veggies with dips, and yogurt with granola.

Other natural remedies

Nourish your muscles with amino acids

You don't have to be an athlete or a weight lifter to benefit from amino acid supplements. Promising research suggests these building blocks of protein could help older people maintain muscle and improve their fitness as they age.

Sarcopenia, the loss of muscle mass that comes with aging, contributes to falls, frailty, fractures, and loss of independence. It also increases your risk of heart disease and metabolic syndrome, a combination of risk factors for diabetes and heart disease. Experts think part of the problem is failing to stay active as you age, compounded by not eating enough protein.

That's where amino acids come in. These compounds are the building blocks of protein. Your body can make some of them, but others must come from the food you eat. Athletes, body builders, and dieters sometimes take amino acid supplements, but small studies suggest seniors may benefit from them, too.

Fend off falls. Researchers gave 2.4 grams (g) of the amino acid beta-alanine to 12 older men and women, while 14 others received fake pills, called placebos. After 90 days, eight people taking beta-alanine got a fitness boost, compared to just three people taking the placebo. The results also suggest the supplement could help prevent falls among older adults and help them live longer on their own.

Stay fit on bed rest. A supplement combining amino acids and carbohydrate preserved muscle mass in people during four weeks of bed rest.

Carbohydrates trigger your body to release insulin. If you also have plenty of amino acids in your system, which is the case after eating protein-filled food or taking an amino acid supplement, then insulin stimulates your cells to absorb those amino acids and begin building protein.

Getting these nutrients in combination seems to have a greater effect than getting them separately. Experts think these nutrients could slow muscle loss in people who can't move or have trouble exercising, although the supplement did not fully preserve muscle strength. That probably requires exercise.

Weigh whey protein. A general protein supplement may build more muscle in the elderly than individual amino acid supplements, according to new research. Again, insulin may hold the key.

Researchers gave one group of seniors 15 g of a whey protein supplement and another a pure amino acid supplement. The whey protein led to a bigger spike in insulin levels and greater muscle gain in the long run. Experts say the bump in insulin levels combined with the extra shot of amino acids found naturally in whey protein stimulated more muscle building.

More protein isn't always better. Getting too much protein or amino acids can harm your kidneys and potentially fuel the growth of dormant tumors in your gut and liver. Besides that, protein alone probably won't stop sarcopenia. You may also need to add in aerobic exercise, such as walking, and resistance exercises, like lifting weights. Talk to your doctor if you're worried about losing muscle, and discuss whether a regimen of supplements and exercise could help.

Safer way to ease aches and pains

Nonsteroidal anti-inflammatory drugs (NSAIDs), which include ibuprofen and naproxen, can help relieve your back pain and neck pain, but potentially at the expense of your health. Research links these potent drugs to ulcers, bleeding, heart attacks, and even death. Maybe it's time to put down the pills and pick up some fish oil, an effective and safe alternative.

Numerous studies show fish oil supplements relieve the painful, tender joints and morning stiffness of rheumatoid arthritis. Now, University of Pittsburgh researchers have found that omega-3 fatty acids, the anti-inflammatory compound in fish oil, may treat neck and back pain, too.

Researchers asked 125 people with nonsurgical neck or back pain to take a total of 1,200 milligrams (mg) a day of fish oil supplements, which are loaded with omega-3. After two-and-a-half months:

■ six out of 10 sufferers were able to stop taking NSAIDs for pain.

■ six in 10 people said both their overall pain and joint pain had improved.

■ nearly nine in 10 said they would continue taking the supplements.

Fish oil boasts two types of omega-3 — EPA and DHA — which squash the production of inflammation-causing compounds within your body. It also tends to thin the blood, so talk to your doctor before trying these supplements if you have a bleeding disorder or take blood thinners, such as Coumadin (warfarin) or heparin. If you decide to give them a try, divide your total daily dose into two or three small doses and take them throughout the day with meals.

Quiet legs naturally

Valerian, an herb used for centuries as a safe sleep aid, may offer an alternative treatment to restless legs syndrome. Drugs currently prescribed for RLS can leave you with day-time sleepiness and rebound insomnia, and they may stop working over time. But a recent study showed that taking 800 milligrams (mg) of valerian daily for eight weeks improved RLS symptoms and decreased daytime sleepiness.

Herbs to curb back pain

Two out of every three American adults will have back pain during their lifetimes, and the problem becomes more common with age as your spine begins to wear and tear from everyday living. When chronic back pain flares up, try a promising herbal remedy such as devil's claw or white willow bark, instead of risky drugs.

Nonsteroidal anti-inflammatory drugs (NSAIDs), like ibuprofen and Celebrex, are easy solutions, but their potential side effects, including stomach bleeding, ulcers, and heart problems, make them risky in managing pain long-term. Two herbal treatments may beat back pain with fewer side effects.

Devil's claw. Don't let the name scare you. There's nothing sinister about this pain-relieving herb. Natives in the steppes of South Africa use the root tubers of *Harpagophytum procumbens*, or devil's claw, to treat muscle and skeleton complaints, among other conditions. In fact, the European Scientific Cooperative on Phytotherapy recommends it for relieving lower back pain and the aches of osteoarthritis.

This herb packs real pain-relieving and anti-inflammatory properties, and lab studies suggest devil's claw puts a stop to the domino effect that leads to inflammation in your body. Taking at least 50 milligrams (mg) of a harpagoside supplement daily seemed to ease joint and back pain in studies. Harpagoside is a major component of *Harpagophytum procumbens*.

Talk to your doctor before trying devil's claw. People taking blood-thinning medications or with a history of bleeding problems, ulcers, or stroke should be especially careful with this herb. Stop taking the herb two weeks before undergoing surgery, medical tests, or any dental procedure that could involve bleeding, and wait awhile before starting them again.

White willow bark. This herb, also known as *Salix alba*, has worked as well as or better than conventional back pain medications in studies, including the class of NSAIDs known as COX-2 inhibitors. It's also cheaper.

A review of the research showed that taking 240 mg of *Salix alba* a day in the form of salicin relieved pain about as well as 12.5 mg of the now banned COX-2 inhibitor Vioxx. Like aspirin, the herb relieves pain and keeps blood platelets from sticking together. Avoid it if you are allergic to aspirin, and take it with caution if you suffer from digestive problems, such as ulcers.

Most of the research on both of these herbal pain relievers comes from only short-term trials, up to six weeks long, and about half the researchers had a personal stake in the results. Experts want to see more and better studies before recommending these herbal cures. Discuss them with your doctor before trying them if you think they might work for you.

Iron out itchy, twitchy legs

Bedtime is anything but relaxing when you have restless legs syndrome (RLS). Between the strong urge to move your legs and the uncomfortable creepy-crawly sensations, it's tough to get a good night's sleep. Finding relief, however, may not be as hard. In some cases, the right supplements can help.

Those itching, pulling, fidgety sensations usually start or become worse in the evenings and when you rest, especially if you're lying down. You're not alone. As many as one in four people over age 65 struggles with RLS. It often runs in families, with women more likely to get it than men, and the condition becomes more common with age.

RLS involves more than age, gender, or genetics. It's also linked to anemia, or iron deficiency. In fact, up to 30 percent of people with low iron levels may develop RLS. Three out of four people with RLS may have an iron shortage, as well.

The link is hard to ignore. Experts suspect some people may have trouble processing iron. When your iron levels drop, your body can't produce enough of the brain chemical dopamine. A shortage of this crucial chemical could be the culprit behind RLS for some sufferers.

Research supports this theory. Studies show iron supplements can significantly improve RLS symptoms in people who are iron deficient, but not in people who have normal iron levels. Ask your doctor to test your iron levels with a blood test. If your levels come back as less than 50 micrograms per liter, then getting more iron every day may help.

Your doctor may suggest eating more iron-rich foods, then recommend supplements if that doesn't help. Typically, people with iron-deficiency anemia take 200 milligrams (mg) of elemental iron divided into two or three doses a day, but 65 mg of daily iron may be enough to resolve RLS.

Don't start the supplements without talking to your doctor and getting your blood levels tested. Overdosing on iron is a real risk and serious business. The supplements can have side effects, including dark feces, nausea, vomiting, and diarrhea. If your doctor approves, take the pills between meals with a full glass of water, and store them in a cool, dark, dry place — not your bathroom medicine cabinet.

Healthful living

Amazing alternative therapies ease chronic pain

Chronic pain can make your life miserable, but so can drugs and risky surgeries. When you strain a muscle, the pain eventually goes away, but chronic pain never leaves. That's why doctors prescribe so many painkillers for back pain, neck pain, arthritis, fibromyalgia, and similar conditions every year. Yet, drugs are not always the answer. More than a dozen alternative therapies may ease chronic pain when drugs can't. Even better, alternative therapies are becoming very common as more hospitals offer them. Before you agree to surgery, talk with your doctor about trying safe and effective alternative therapies like these.

Chiropractic. Your spinal column has 33 bony vertebrae. Hundreds of nerves branch off the spine through openings in these vertebrae.

Chiropractors believe tiny misalignments in the vertebrae, called subluxations, can pinch these nerves. This may prevent the body parts served by the nerves from functioning correctly. By adjusting your vertebrae to eliminate subluxations, chiropractors relieve the pressure on your nerves, so your body can heal.

Studies suggest chiropractic treatment may naturally ease back and neck muscle pain, migraines, and osteoarthritis without the side effects you'd get from drugs. If you decide to seek chiropractic treatment for osteoarthritis, remember that chiropractic manipulation of weak or damaged joints may lead to trouble. Find a chiropractor who has regularly worked on people with arthritis and be sure to tell her you have arthritis.

Massage. Several studies report that massage can temporarily ease low back pain. In fact, one review suggests massage may help people diagnosed with "nonspecific" low back pain — the kind that lasts one to three months and isn't caused by another health problem. Massage may be particularly good for this kind of back pain when combined with exercise and health education. For neck or shoulder pain, massage that targets local areas of the body may be better than full body massage.

Before you try massage, check the credentials of any massage therapist you consider. Look for a massage therapist who is licensed, registered, or certified by your state. Most states require this. Also, check for the Nationally Certified in Therapeutic Massage and Bodywork (NCTMB) designation.

Acupuncture. According to a medical report, a 49-year-old woman with several serious health problems had such severe knee pain and insomnia she couldn't fully participate in her medical treatment. So in addition to her regular medical care, her doctors prescribed a course of acupuncture. Not only did acupuncture substantially improve her sleep and knee pain, but the results lasted at least 15 weeks beyond her last acupuncture session.

Acupuncture needles may sound scary, but they're as thin as a strand of hair. Acupuncturists temporarily insert these needles at the specific points on the body believed to relieve pain. They believe this restores the proper flow of energy through the body, helping you heal. Studies suggest acupuncture may help low back pain as much or more than standard treatment. And a Mayo Clinic study found that acupuncture significantly reduces pain, fatigue, and anxiety in people with mild to moderate fibromyalgia.

Alexander technique. The Alexander technique teaches how to properly coordinate the body to release harmful tension, relieve pain, reduce fatigue, and to improve coordination, balance, and health. British researchers say this technique may ease back pain by reducing muscle spasms, releasing tension in the spine, building up postural muscles, and boosting flexibility. In fact, a study found that the Alexander technique was better at reducing back pain than massage therapy or exercise alone. And here's a cost-saving tip — six lessons plus exercise were nearly as effective as 24 lessons.

Stress management. Stress may not cause pain, but it can make pain worse. Exercise and listening to music can help, but so can these mind-body techniques.

- meditation — concentrating on your breathing or a single word to quiet tensions

- guided imagery — visualizing a relaxing place or event

- relaxation — easing tension through techniques like controlled breathing

Not every case of chronic pain, especially back and neck pain, are candidates for alternative therapies. Work with your doctor to find out the cause of your pain to make sure you don't cause more harm than good. Seek medical help quickly if you experience a sudden, unexplained backache, weakness in your legs, sudden problems with bladder or bowel function, or numbness in the anal or genital regions.

Everyday ways to prevent back and neck aches

Little things can make a big difference. Making a few simple changes in your daily routine can help you avoid back and neck pain.

Forget what you've heard. Sitting up straight isn't really good for your back. Neither is hunching over your desk. Instead, a new study from Scotland suggests that sitting while leaning back puts less strain on the lumbar spine and retains its natural shape. To sit in this position, use a comfy recliner or tilt your office chair back so you can lean back about halfway to lying down. When you need to sit up for desk work, raise your chair so your thighs are a little diagonal when your spine is vertical.

Stop purse pain. Oversized purses may be stylish, but they can cause back pain, shoulder stiffness, headaches, and stiff necks. This happens because the purse's weight pulls down on your shoulder, straining your neck and the nerves that exit the neck and line your shoulder. To ease this strain, clean out your purse every week. Reorganize the remaining contents so all the pockets get used. This helps distribute weight more evenly. Clean out your wallet too. Carry only the cash and the credit cards you need. Also, don't always carry your bag on the same shoulder. Alternate between shoulders or cradle the purse in front of you in both arms.

Get a headset. Don't cradle your phone or cell phone between your ear and neck. Consider getting a headset or speakerphone if you need to talk with your hands free.

Sit back in your seat while driving. If your seat can't give you enough back support, roll up a blanket or some towels to tuck behind your lower back. For added comfort, use cruise control whenever possible and shift your weight from time to time.

Beware wallet sciatica. An overstuffed wallet can cause pain in your rear end, back, leg, and hip because it puts pressure on your sciatic nerve. Clean out your overstuffed wallet, switch to an ultra-thin wallet, carry your wallet in a side or front pants pocket, or carry it in a briefcase.

Compute comfortably. Laptops make you scrunch. When you use your laptop, you probably either hunch your neck and head over because the monitor is too low or you hold your shoulders and hands oddly because the keyboard is too high. This can cause pain in your neck, shoulders, and back. Use one or more of the following to help position your monitor at eye level and your keyboard at elbow level — laptop stands, external keyboards, keyboard tray, external mouse, or a docking station.

Spend time with friends to feel better

Suffering from chronic pain? Get by with a little help from your friends. A Spanish study found that strong social support may help ease pain and the depression that often comes with it. That same support also seemed to encourage people to take a more active role in dealing with pain, resulting in more relief.

Tailor your exercise to type of pain

Staying fit and being physically active can prevent chronic pain. But once you're laid low with an ongoing painful condition, like back pain or fibromyalgia, you need to find relief.

A review of 20 studies found that exercise is effective at preventing back pain while other tactics — like shoe inserts, lumbar back supports, and reduced lifting programs — were not effective. Experts think regular physical activities like walking or biking may help prevent back pain because they strengthen your back and abdominal muscles.

If you already have back or neck pain, weight lifting may be even better, studies suggest. A Canadian study found that 16 weeks of weight lifting improved back pain far more than 16 weeks of aerobic exercises, like walking on a treadmill. Aerobics only strengthens the lower body. Weight lifting strengthens the whole body and may reduce the fatigue caused by daily activities. Tai chi and meditation may also ease back pain.

A study of office workers found that neck pain can be helped by either neck exercises that work against gravity or strength training with resistance bands. If your doctor says you have simple neck pain from too much desk work, try this easy stretch. Relax your arms at your sides. Raise your shoulders up toward your ears, pull them back while raised, wait a few seconds, and then let your shoulders relax. Do 10 of these twice a day.

If your chronic pain comes from fibromyalgia, try aerobic exercise instead. London researchers found that aerobic exercise helped reduce fibromyalgia pain in just three months. Experts recommend graded exercise, meaning you gradually increase the time you spend exercising. Experiment with walking, swimming, or using a treadmill or stationary bike.

#1 way to feel younger than your years

You may have trouble lifting your groceries or even lifting yourself out of a chair as you get older. But if you start lifting weights, you may be able to reverse the muscle loss that comes with aging.

Sarcopenia is a gradual loss of muscle strength and muscle mass as you age. This condition affects nearly 45 percent of Americans age 60 and up. People with severe sarcopenia can't rise from a chair or get out of bed without help. Some may even have trouble walking, climbing stairs, or going to the bathroom. These problems interfere with the daily activities of living and deprive many older adults of their independence.

As if that's not enough, sarcopenia contributes to falls, obesity, type 2 diabetes, and perhaps to heart failure and chronic obstructive pulmonary disease. Fortunately, you can slow the progress of sarcopenia and keep more of your strength for longer with simple weight lifting exercises.

Fight your body's aging process. Studies show that men and women start losing muscle strength and mass around age 40 and lose another 10 percent with each passing decade. That means you could be down to 50 percent of your original strength and muscle mass by age 90. Start weight lifting now and you may do more than just prevent future muscle loss. You may start getting your strength back.

According to a small University of Alabama study, women in their 60s and 70s who did four months of weight lifting improved their strength by up to 50 percent. They also increased their walking speed and improved their ability to do daily tasks, like carrying groceries. Scientists think weight lifting may work because it actually makes changes inside your muscle cells.

Make your muscles younger. Each of your cells contains energy producers called mitochondria. As you age, the mitochondria start malfunctioning, possibly because the genes inside them stop working properly. Scientists suspect this may impact your muscles and help cause sarcopenia. In fact, when researchers compared the strength of healthy, older adults to younger adults, they discovered that older adults' muscle strength was 59 percent lower. After six months of weight lifting twice a week, the older adults' strength increased by 50 percent — partially reversing years of dwindling muscle strength.

Researchers also compared muscle fiber samples from both younger and older adults. Samples taken before weight training suggested older adults' mitochondria had fewer fully functioning genes than mitochondria from younger adults. After weight training, many of the genes from older adults started working again, making their mitochondria and muscles more like those of younger adults. That's like rejuvenating your muscle tissue so it actually becomes younger. If that's what six months of weight lifting can do, imagine how much you'll benefit if you do it for life. Who knows, you might even end up with the strength of someone half your age.

Reap extra benefits. This doesn't mean you should start lifting heavy weights every day. Instead, get your doctor's permission and then start slowly. Experts recommend that beginners only commit one hour a week to weight lifting. If you gradually work up to two or three hours a week, you may not only regain strength and muscle but also reap bonus benefits like these.

- Fight diabetes. Weight lifting and moderate weight loss helped older people with type 2 diabetes improve blood sugar control, boost muscle strength, and raise lean body mass, an Australian study found. The trick is to do high-intensity, progressive weight lifting. High intensity means you lift weights that are 70 percent of the most weight you can lift, and progressive means you add more weight as you grow stronger.

- Lower your blood pressure. A review of studies suggests four or more weeks of weight lifting can lower your blood pressure. Stronger muscles from weight lifting help bring your blood pressure down by reducing the demands your daily activities make on your heart.

- Ease arthritis pain. Studies show weight lifting strengthens muscles. Making your muscles stronger may help protect your joints from even more damage.

- Improve your memory. Physical activity such as walking and weight lifting may help improve memory and mental abilities in older adults with memory problems.

- Stop osteoporosis. Weight lifting puts tension on both muscle and bone, making your body increase the density and strength of your bones.

- Improve your posture. Strength training also improves your posture, coordination, and balance, while helping you burn fat.

Improve workouts with caffeine

Drink coffee before exercising, and you may push yourself harder. Enjoy another cup afterward, and you'll build up fuel reserves for your next workout. Either way, caffeine can enhance your exercise program. Caffeine before a workout may help you exercise harder or longer because it reduces exercise pain. You feel less pain because caffeine blocks adenosine, a chemical that helps with pain processing.

Caffeine may also help your muscles recover after an intense workout. The compound glycogen is the fuel your muscles use up during intense exercise. But an Australian study reports that elite cyclists who consumed both carbohydrates and caffeine after a tough workout had 66 percent higher levels of glycogen four hours after working out.

Apparently, caffeine helps move glucose from food into your muscles where it becomes your fresh supply of glycogen. When your muscles are low in glycogen, they feel tired and achy.

Shape up successfully at home

Forget the gym with its muscle-bound men and perfectly toned women. You can stay at home and use simple household items to make an exercise program part of your life.

■ Tone your muscles with hand-size bottles, soft drink cans, soup cans, or vegetable cans. They make good hand weights for arm exercises. To add weight as you grow stronger, drop two or more cans or bottles into a sock and tie it off. Do the same with a second sock. Books and tools can also be good weights.

- Strengthen your grip by squeezing a tennis ball.

- Make your own ankle weights. Fill two socks with dry sand or dry rice. Tie them shut, but leave enough room in the toe to fasten the weight around your ankles.

- Fill two medium-size plastic buckets with water or sand. Use these for biceps curls and shoulder exercises. Be careful not to spill the water or sand.

- Stairs in your home or apartment building can help your workout, too. Do calf raises or simply walk up and down the steps.

- Use 5- or 10-pound bags of sugar or potatoes to do chest presses.

- Do lateral raises holding small water or soft drink bottles.

- Rest your calves on the couch or a kitchen chair to help with crunches. Use the couch, a counter, or even your coffee table to brace your arms for dips.

Whether you choose to work out at home or in a gym, keep these tips in mind.

- If you do aerobics, weights, and stretching on the same day, do the aerobics first, then weights, and then stretching. Weights before aerobics can tire muscles. And it's best to stretch after a workout, when your muscles are warmed up.

- If you are over age 60, aim for just two weight lifting sessions a week, with at least one day off in between. Your muscles need at least a day to recover.

- Stretch each muscle group at least two or three times a week.

The truth about juiced-up waters

It's important to stay hydrated while exercising — but don't expect an extra boost of nutrition from enhanced bottled water beverages.

These costly waters are pumped up with vitamins, herbs, antioxidants, and fiber, but at least one expert says enhanced waters may not contain enough nutrients to do you much good. What's more, these waters may also deliver artificial sweeteners, hidden caffeine, or lots of sugar, which pumps up the calories.

Some enhanced waters have up to 130 calories a bottle, nearly as much as some soft drinks. At least one vitamin water has 8 teaspoons of sugar — as much as some chocolate bars. So skip the enhanced waters. Drink green tea or tap water instead and get your nutrients from food.

9 ways to prevent falls

Fear of falling keeps many seniors from participating in activities or leaving home — but your home has its own share of hazards. Follow these tips to make your home environment safer.

■ Don't grip the shower door or towel bar to help you get in and out of the shower or up from the toilet. Regular bathroom fixtures like these aren't built to take your weight. Instead, install sturdy grab bars.

■ Slippery or poorly lit stairs make missteps more likely. Put nonskid treads on the stairs and make sure the stairway is well lit.

- Loose rugs and mats that slide can be like stepping on a banana peel. If you must use mats and throw rugs, only buy those with nonskid backing. Tape or tack down throw rugs and mats you already own.

- Wet or waxed floors are a slippery hazard. Place a rubber mat near the sink or wear rubber-soled shoes in the kitchen.

- Turn on lights or light your expected path with night lights if you sometimes get up during the night. Make sure the lights are bright enough to clearly light your way.

According to the Centers for Disease Control and Prevention, more than 21,000 older adults are treated in hospital emergency rooms every year for falls associated with their pets — especially dogs. These falls may occur while chasing or walking your pet or because you trip over toys or a food bowl. But this doesn't mean you should give up your pets. Instead, use these tips.

- Take your dog to obedience classes to learn self-control when walking on the leash.

- Pick up pet toys — and any other clutter — regularly.

- Put your pet outside or in another area of the house when cleaning or carrying in groceries.

- Discourage pets from lying or sleeping near beds or chairs.

Put a positive spin on dizziness

Dizziness makes you feel unsteady and lightheaded, as if you're spinning. Not surprisingly, dizziness also makes you more likely to fall. Often, a medical condition is to blame, but some everyday situations can also cause dizziness. Either way, simple steps like these can help prevent dizziness from disrupting your balance.

Get more sleep. A study of older women found that getting five hours of sleep or less raises your risk of falls. Aim for at least seven hours of sleep each night.

Manage low blood pressure. Situations that cause a temporary drop in your blood pressure may lead to dizziness and fainting. For example, some people have postural (orthostatic) hypotension. That means your blood pressure plummets when you stand up from sitting or lying down. That may cause dizziness, blurry vision, lightheadedness, and fainting. Postural hypotension may be caused by diabetes, dehydration, prolonged bed rest, or heart problems. You may also get this low blood pressure from getting overheated, which can happen during summer outdoor work or if you take a steamy shower without enough ventilation.

If you have postural hypotension, drink liquids regularly to keep hydrated and avoid getting overheated. If this low blood pressure is caused by a medical condition, talk to your doctor about how to manage this problem.

Beware of zinc overdose. A recent report found that several people who used two or more tubes of denture cream a week developed brain and nerve problems because they were getting a zinc overdose from the cream. Symptoms included balance problems and weakness in their arms and legs. These symptoms can raise your risk of falls. If you use more than one tube of denture cream every three weeks, you may experience the same problems as the people in the report. Tell your doctor and your dentist immediately.

But don't forget that medical conditions may also cause dizziness. For example, benign paroxysmal positional vertigo (BPPV) is an inner ear problem that's the most common form of vertigo. Vertigo is dizziness that makes you feel as if you or your surroundings are moving. BPPV is triggered by calcium carbonate crystals that break loose in your inner ear. Fortunately, your doctor can perform a quick and painless treatment called the Epley maneuver. This maneuver puts the crystals back where they belong and stops the dizziness for most people. You'll get the best results when this is done with help from a professional so ask your doctor about it.

If you need frequent Epley maneuver treatments, ask your doctor about DizzyFIX. This is a prescription product newly approved by the FDA that may guide you through the Epley maneuver at home.

Dizziness may also be a sign of a more serious condition. If you have dizzy spells that last minutes or hours accompanied by a fast, fluttering heartbeat and shortness of breath, this may be a sign of arrhythmia, an irregular heartbeat. Get medical help right away.

Other conditions that can contribute to dizziness include vision problems like cataracts, wax in the ear, hearing problems, inner ear disorders such as Meniere's disease, strokes, and drug side effects. If dizziness is a problem for you, talk with your doctor to find out what's causing it and how to fix it. Meanwhile, take extra precautions like these to manage dizziness and avoid falls.

- Sit on the edge of your bed for a minute before standing in the morning.

- Store often-used items between waist- and eye-level and use a reaching device to pick up items off the floor to avoid bending down.

- Try waist-high compression stockings if dizziness occurs when you stand up too quickly.

Easy way to better balance

Half of older adults think they'll be less likely to fall if they cut back on their level of physical activity. But experts say the opposite may be true. Many exercises help improve your stability and balance as you age.

Tai chi. This is an easy, slow motion exercise that anyone can benefit from no matter what their age. You simply follow a pattern of flowing movements through various poses and stances. The motions are gentle and graceful so you don't need strong muscles or super flexibility. That's why older women may find it easy to stick with this kind of exercise. But gentle doesn't mean ineffective.

Research suggests tai chi has been proven to improve balance, prevent falls, and increase physical performance skills. An Australian study of obese older adults with type 2 diabetes found that tai chi was just as effective at improving balance and mobility as gentle stretching and calisthenics.

According to Harvard research, a one-hour tai chi session three times a week was just as good as brisk walking for improving balance, flexibility, and knee strength in older women. But tai chi also helped women improve on two measures of aerobic fitness and heart health. That's why tai chi may also be just as good a workout for your heart as brisk walking.

Yoga. Like tai chi, yoga is a low-impact exercise, but both these exercises improve your balance and strength. That's why studies suggest yoga and tai chi may reduce your risk of falls by almost 50 percent.

One type of yoga called Iyengar yoga lets you use props to help with poses. A preliminary Temple University study of women over age 65 suggests this yoga can help improve stability and balance. After just nine weeks of yoga classes, the study participants had a faster stride, increased flexibility in their legs, and more confidence in their walking and balance. The researchers say this improved balance and stability may help reduce the danger of falls.

Stretching. But if taking yoga or tai chi classes isn't for you, consider gardening or line dancing to improve your balance — or simply do stretches at home. You can start with these.

- Plantar flexion stretch. Hold on to a chair or table for balance. Slowly stand on tiptoe, count to two, and lower your heels. Repeat up to 15 times, rest for a minute, and then repeat another eight to 15 times.

- Knee flexion stretch. Hold on to a chair or table for balance. Bend one knee so you slowly raise your foot behind you, count to two, and slowly lower your foot. Rest for a few seconds and repeat with the other leg. Repeat this exercise, switching from one leg to the other, until you've done up to 15 repetitions with each leg.

- Hip flexion stretch. While gripping a chair or table for balance, slowly raise one knee in front of you so it is at the same height as your hip. Count to two and slowly lower your foot to the ground. Do the same with the other leg. Repeat this exercise, switching from one leg to the other, until you've done up to 15 repetitions with each leg.

Smart strategies for sound sleep

Sleep deprived? You're not alone. Insomnia affects about 60 million Americans each year. Find out how to get all the sleep you need just by making some simple lifestyle changes.

Sometimes your own busy mind is the biggest barrier between you and sleep. Fortunately, cognitive behavioral therapy (CBT) may help you stop worrying and start sleeping. In formal CBT, a professional works with you to change the behaviors that prevent sleep by changing unhealthy beliefs and misconceptions about sleep. People treated with either CBT or a combination of CBT and the sleep drug, zolpidem, took less time to fall asleep, woke up less during the night, and generally slept better, a Canadian study found. Of the people who took zolpidem and CBT, those who stopped the drug after six weeks fared better than those who continued taking it.

If your insurer doesn't cover CBT sessions, you can expect to pay up to $150 a session for the five sessions needed to ease your insomnia. To find a cognitive behavioral therapist, get a recommendation from your sleep doctor or visit *www.academyofct.org*.

But you may not need professional help if you take a good look at how you approach your bedroom and sleep. Tour your bedroom to figure out which things help you sleep and which ones are sleep-blockers.

- Clock. Is it helping you set a regular sleep schedule or distressing you each time you check it during the night? Position the clock so it's hard to see from your bed. Worrying over time just makes falling asleep tougher.

- Television. Do you use it near bedtime to watch shows that trigger strong emotions or tension? Tape your favorite shows and watch them earlier in the evening.

- Lamp. Is the light dim and soothing or bright and harsh? Bright light at night tells your body to wake up. Use night lights for hallways and bathrooms and a low-intensity lamp for your bedroom.

- Computer. Do you use it to play soothing CDs or for tense tasks like figuring out your finances or playing video games? One study suggests that using the computer before bed may make you feel less rested the next day even if you haven't gotten less sleep. Listening to slow, relaxing music before bed may help you sleep, research shows.

- Bed. Is it a comfy, inviting place for snoozing or do you use it for late-day naps, television-watching, and other things that may sabotage sleep? Use your bed only for slumber and sex. Keep naps short and don't take them after 3 p.m.

- Bathroom. Is this where you take evening baths or where you make frequent toilet stops during the night? Taking a bath right before bedtime may make you more alert. Try that hot bath about an hour and a half to two hours before bedtime. This helps you fall asleep more easily and stay asleep. Also, avoid fluids before bed so you won't visit the bathroom during the night.

- Thermostat or fan. Do you adjust these to keep your room comfortable during the night? You'll sleep better if you keep your bedroom cool, not warm and stuffy.

- Weights or exercise equipment. Do you use these to exercise during the day or close to bedtime? Exercising close to bedtime may make you more energetic, so exercise shortly before dinner instead.

Now that you know how to stop sabotaging your sleep, use these bonus tips to make falling asleep even easier.

- Go to bed and wake up at the same time every day.

- Do only relaxing things during the half-hour before bedtime.

- Eat a light dinner four to five hours before bedtime. A large meal may interfere with sleep.

- Spend a half hour in the sun early in the day.

- Use soothing sounds to sleep more soundly. A study suggests that white noise, similar to the sounds of a fan or humidifier, may help you sleep.

Simple device guides you to dreamland

See the light, and stop relying on sleeping pills. The NightWave Sleep Assistant is a safe, natural product that may put an end to your sleep problems. Here's how it works.

NightWave shines a soft, blue light that alternately brightens and dims. You inhale as the light brightens and exhale as it dims. This helps guide you through a series of deep breathing exercise patterns that should gradually relax your body and mind and help you fall asleep. You can set the NightWave to automatically shut off after 7 minutes or 25 minutes.

Expect to pay around $60 for a regular NightWave or $70 for the travel version. For more information, visit *www.nightwave.com* or call toll free 866-260-7021.

Run away from restless legs

Distractions or poor sleep habits aren't the only things that keep you up at night. Restless legs syndrome (RLS), which affects up to 15 percent of adults in the United States, can also interfere with your sleep. When you have RLS, you get a disturbing sensation in your legs and the irresistible urge to move them. Ironically, the solution may be to move your legs more during the day. Exercise can help treat — and even prevent — RLS.

Many people who have RLS also have periodic limb movement disorder (PLMD), a condition that causes your legs to jerk involuntarily during the night. PLMD may lead to poor quality sleep, daytime drowsiness, and reduced alertness. Exercise can help decrease those nightly leg movements, a small Brazilian study found. The study compared two groups of sedentary adults with PLMD. One group did a single, intense workout (acute group), while another group completed 72 exercise sessions (chronic group).

Both groups had fewer leg movements during the night. However, the acute group also became less likely to wake during the night, spent more of the night sleeping, and increased their REM sleep, the kind of sleep crucial to your learning processes. Meanwhile, the chronic group fell asleep faster and spent more of the night sleeping than they did before they'd begun exercising.

Even if you don't have PLMD or RLS yet, exercise can help you lose weight and narrow your waist — and that may help prevent RLS. A new study found that people with a body mass index (BMI) score over 30 were nearly 1.5 times more likely to have RLS than those with a BMI under 23. What's more, people with the highest waist measurements were 1.5 times more likely to have RLS than people with the smallest waist measurements.

More research is needed to confirm whether keeping a low BMI score and small waist size could help prevent RLS. Some studies suggest that people who are obese have fewer receptors in their brains for the natural chemical messenger called dopamine. Since low brain levels of dopamine are thought to play a key role in RLS, this may help explain how obesity and RLS could be connected.

3 steps to better breathing

About 12 million Americans have chronic obstructive pulmonary disease (COPD), which includes emphysema and chronic bronchitis. If you are one of them, you can manage your symptoms and live more comfortably with these tips.

Learn to play the harmonica. This could be the most fun way to improve your breathing. Little holes run the length of the harmonica and each one plays a different note. To play the harmonica, you must blow through pursed lips to keep from playing too many notes at once. This pursed lip breathing exercises muscles in the diaphragm, which leads to easier breathing. Experts say playing the harmonica may help people with emphysema, chronic bronchitis, and asthma. If you'd like to learn to improve your breathing with a harmonica, check for classes at patient support groups or nearby hospitals. Or order the book and CD program *Harmonica for Fun & Health* from *www.harmonicamasterclass.com*.

If playing the harmonica isn't for you, try pursed lip breathing exercises on your own. When you feel short of breath, sit and breathe in through your nose then out through your mouth. As soon as you feel able, try to blow out for longer than you breathe in. It may help to purse your lips each time you breathe out, while tightening your abdominal muscles to help you let air out more slowly and fully.

As you feel better, start breathing through your nose and try to breathe slowly from your diaphragm, a muscle located between your chest cavity and your abdominal cavity. Your diaphragm contracts and moves downward to allow your lungs to expand when you inhale, and it relaxes when you exhale.

Watch your waistline. A big stomach can press in on your diaphragm, the main muscle you use for breathing, and make it more difficult for you to take a breath. In fact, studies from Scotland, Canada, and France have all found that a bigger waist means poorer lung function. The French study even suggests that a waist measurement of 35 inches for women and 40 inches for men is enough to affect your breathing. If your weight has crept up over the years, consider slimming down to breathe easier.

Get your shots. Reduced lung capacity not only raises your risk of pneumonia but also your risk of complications from the flu and pneumonia. Talk with your doctor about getting a flu shot and ask whether you should get vaccinated for pneumonia, too.

Medical alternatives

Get relief without the grief

It hurts, plain and simple. You've tried exercise, stretching, rest, massage, heat packs, and guided imagery and gotten some relief. But right now it hurts, and you're going to have to take medication to ease the pain. There's nothing necessarily wrong with that, as long as you're careful and informed about how medication affects your body.

Understand body basics. As you age, your body changes. So does its ability to absorb, distribute, break down, and eliminate drugs. Changes in your body weight, digestive system, circulatory system, liver, and kidneys can all affect how drugs work and the dosage you need. For example, your liver and kidneys work more slowly as you get older, so drugs stay in your system longer. A lower dose may have the same effect. On the other hand, if you have trouble absorbing a drug, you may need a higher dose.

These body changes increase the risk of dangerous drug interactions. One drug may cause another not to work as well or make it stronger than it should be. To be safe, ask your doctor to start you off with the lowest dose, then increase it as necessary.

Explain the pain. The better you can describe your pain, the more it will help your doctor make the right decisions. Keep a pain diary, noting when and how you feel pain. Is it burning, aching, throbbing, sharp, or dull? Be specific. You may want to rate your pain on a scale of 1 to 10. What makes it feel worse or better? How does it affect your mood, sleep, or other activities? Work with your doctor to set pain relief goals.

Know your options. Your best bet for mild to moderate muscle and bone pain is acetaminophen. It's the top choice of the

American Geriatrics Society — but it's also a pretty weak painkiller. Although it's safe and effective for most people, too much can lead to liver damage and death. Be careful about combining medications that contain acetaminophen, such as pain relievers and cough and cold remedies. Do not use if you drink heavily or have a liver disorder.

Nonsteroidal anti-inflammatory drugs (NSAIDs), including aspirin, naproxen, and ibuprofen, ease pain and fight inflammation. But they come with many risks for older people with chronic pain. They can cause life-threatening ulcers and stomach bleeding, increase the risk of heart attack or stroke, make high blood pressure worse, damage your kidneys, and interact with other drugs. Use only for a short period of time under a doctor's care.

Be aware of the pros and cons. Opioids, including morphine, oxycodone, codeine, and hydrocodone, are very powerful drugs derived from opium that change the way you perceive pain. They may cause drowsiness and constipation and should not be mixed with alcohol, antihistamines, barbiturates, or benzodiazepines. They can also be addictive. However, for older people, they may be safer than NSAIDs.

Some drugs pair an opioid with acetaminophen, aspirin, or ibuprofen. The two ingredients work to relieve your pain in different ways, and the smaller doses of each mean less risk of side effects. Antidepressants are often prescribed for lower back pain, but recent evidence suggests they may not be effective. Here are a few more things worth considering.

■ Never change the dose of your pain medication without talking to your doctor.

■ Don't share pain pills with anyone else.

■ Avoid taking multiple medications with the same ingredient at the same time.

- Tell your doctor about all the medicine you take, as well as your alcohol consumption.

- Store drugs in a place where they can't be stolen.

Give restless legs some rest

You may want to avoid sleep-inducing allergy drugs if you have restless legs syndrome (RLS). They can make your symptoms three to four times worse. Johns Hopkins researchers pinpointed the problem — diphenhydramine, the active ingredient in many allergy medications that calms histamine — the substance that makes you sneeze and itch — and brings about sleepiness.

It turns out that people with RLS have a higher number of histamine receptors in the area of the brain involved with the condition. When activated, these receptors affect nerve responses and also spark alertness or wakefulness. This promising discovery could lead to new treatments for RLS. But in the meantime, it's one more path to a restless night.

Shoot down pain with prolotherapy

Just a spoonful of sugar helps the medicine go down. But an injection of a sugar solution may help even more for chronic pain. That's the idea behind prolotherapy.

Chronic pain can be caused by weakened ligaments and tendons. Ligaments connect bone to bone, while tendons connect muscle to bone. Loose ligaments and tendons force muscles to work harder to stabilize joints, leading to muscle pain and spasms. Joints may also become unstable and move in unnatural and painful ways.

Prolotherapy, short for proliferation therapy, involves injections near these sore sites to strengthen the tissue that holds bones and muscles in place. It works in a way completely opposite from anti-inflammatory drugs. While these drugs blunt pain, they may also slow healing. Prolotherapy triggers your body's natural inflammatory response, which promotes the growth and thickening of ligaments and tendons.

Pioneered by Dr. George Hackett in 1939, prolotherapy has been used to treat conditions such as back pain, osteoarthritis, fibromyalgia, plantar fasciitis, sciatica, sports injuries, temporomandibular joint disorder (TMJ), carpal tunnel syndrome, tendonitis, and tension headaches.

Injections may be a simple sugar solution (dextrose) or some other chemical irritant. For best results, you usually need a series of injections every few weeks. Prolotherapy is usually performed by doctors specializing in orthopedics or physical medicine and rehabilitation, chiropractors, and osteopathic doctors. Cost varies, depending on the diagnosis, and the treatment may or may not be covered by insurance. No serious side effects of prolotherapy have been reported, but you may experience some tenderness or stiffness near the injection site after treatment.

So far, clinical studies of prolotherapy have had mixed results. A Canadian study used a modified version of prolotherapy to successfully treat 32 of 36 people with Achilles tendinosis, an overuse injury.

Other studies suggest prolotherapy may work best for osteoarthritis. One review determined that prolotherapy was not an effective treatment for chronic low-back pain by itself. But, when combined with spinal manipulation, exercise, and other treatments, it may reduce pain and disability.

Prolotherapy does boast several individual success stories. For instance, one cyclist recovered from a painful knee injury after three injections over two months. Even actresses and professional football players have benefited from it. Although the scientific evidence remains inconclusive, prolotherapy may be worth a try. It could ease your pain and help you avoid drugs and surgery.

Zap chronic pain with electricity

The next time paying your electric bill causes you financial pain, keep this in mind. Electricity can help relieve chronic pain. Find out more about three electrifying pain therapies.

TENS. Transcutaneous electrical nerve stimulation (TENS) delivers low-voltage electrical current to electrodes placed on your skin. The electrical stimulation blocks the transmission of pain signals to your brain and may even boost the level of feel-good hormones called endorphins.

TENS can be a good short-term fix for back pain. It may also ease pain from arthritis, joint pain, and fibromyalgia. Just clip the pocket-size device to your belt or clothing and attach the electrodes to your back. You'll need to learn how to place the electrodes, adjust the frequency and voltage, and determine the length and intensity of the stimulation.

You usually need a prescription, but the FDA approved some easy-to-use brands — including Medisana, BlueWave, and Well Life — for over-the-counter use. Cost ranges from $100 to $750, and it's covered by many insurance plans. You can also rent a unit. That may be a wise move, since the treatment doesn't work for everyone.

TENS may become less effective as your body gets used to the electrical pulses. Avoid TENS if you have implantable devices, like a defibrillator or pacemaker.

Spinal cord stimulation. In this treatment for chronic pain, a surgically implanted device continuously delivers a low-voltage electrical current to your spinal cord to block the feeling of pain. It works because electrical pulses scramble or block pain signals before they reach your brain.

A Polish review found that spinal cord stimulation reduced pain for those who had "failed back surgery syndrome." It also improved their quality of life. Another study found that about 60 percent of people who received spinal cord stimulation experienced pain reduction or relief when surveyed one to two years after the procedure.

Compared to usual care, spinal cord stimulation is more effective and less costly in the long run. But it does come with a high initial cost. Implants cost about $20,000, and hospital and follow-up costs could double your total bill.

In addition to the expense, there are some other drawbacks. It does not work for everyone, rarely offers complete relief, and comes with several risks. Surgery can lead to allergic reaction, bleeding, infection, paralysis or weakness, spinal fluid leakage, and worsened pain. Technical complications can also occur with the device.

Before getting an implant, you can opt for a trial procedure to see if the technique works for you. When choosing a type of spinal cord stimulator, go with a rechargeable system, which can save you more than $100,000 over your lifetime. It lasts longer than a conventional system and requires fewer surgical procedures to replace the power source.

Electroacupuncture. Consider this a high-tech version of traditional acupuncture. Wires pass low-voltage electrical current through needles to stimulate circulation and spark production of your body's pain-numbing chemicals, such as endorphins, serotonin, and acetylcholine.

This technique could be an effective part of a comprehensive treatment plan for low back pain, fibromyalgia, and several other conditions, including those involving your head and neck, shoulders, elbows, torso, and hips and thighs. Sessions usually last 15 to 30 minutes. In most cases, you'll need a series of treatments. How many depends on the type and seriousness of your injury. Avoid electroacupuncture if you have an irregular heartbeat, high blood pressure, or a pacemaker.

Inhale at your own risk

Using an inhaler for a chronic breathing condition could put you at risk for pneumonia, heart attack, and stroke.

For people with chronic obstructive pulmonary disease (COPD), inhaled corticosteroids, which relieve symptoms like shortness of breath and wheezing, raise pneumonia risk by one-third. This danger is mostly among those taking high doses, people with low lung function, and those who also use a bronchodilator to open airways. But that's not all. People with COPD who used inhaled anticholinergics — drugs to relax the airways — longer than a month were 58 percent more likely to suffer a heart attack, stroke, or death from heart disease.

What can you do? Use the lowest possible steroid dose that works, and get a pneumonia vaccination every five years, experts advise. And make sure you talk to your doctor about the benefits and risks of these inhaled medications.

3 ways to improve the quality of your sleep

Insomnia affects more than half of all seniors. It can also be expensive to treat. Before you turn to costly — and potentially risky — treatments for insomnia, consider this advice.

Prevent pill perils. Sleeping pills may help get you through the night — but they could have serious consequences the next day. University of Toronto researchers determined that people over age 60 are five times more likely to have memory or thinking problems after using sleeping pills. Seniors who use sleeping pills are also nearly three times more likely to suffer a fall and four times more likely to feel tired during the day.

As you age, your metabolism slows down and your body processes drugs more slowly. A sleeping pill that is supposed to last only overnight remains in your body much longer. Daytime grogginess can lead to falls, which can lead to broken bones.

While older sleep aids may cause addiction and withdrawal, newer drugs called nonbenzodiazepines — including zolpidem (Ambien) and eszopiclone (Lunesta) — may spark strange side effects, such as driving, cooking, or eating while asleep.

And that's not all. Make sure the drugs you're taking for other conditions are not causing your insomnia. These include stimulants, antidepressants, corticosteroids, diuretics, anticonvulsants, and some blood-pressure lowering drugs. If you must take these drugs, take them in the morning.

Over-the-counter antihistamines, including diphenhydramine and doxylamine, may help you sleep, but they're not recommended for older people because of their lingering sedating effect. Read labels carefully. You may be taking antihistamines without knowing it. Products like Tylenol PM and Simply Sleep contain 25 milligrams of diphenhydramine in each tablet.

If you do decide to take sleeping pills, take some precautions. Go to bed immediately, since pills can take effect within 15 minutes. Never take more than the maximum dose, mix sleeping pills with alcohol, or try to drive while taking sleeping pills.

Change the way you sleep. Sidestep sleeping pill dangers by changing your sleep habits. Perhaps you're spending too much time in bed, waiting to fall asleep. Simply going to bed a little later can help. If you wake up during the night, get up and read or watch TV in another room until you're sleepy again. Remember, sleeping pills should be a last resort. Practice good sleep hygiene, and you may solve your sleep problem without prescriptions.

Skip the sleep study. Even if you spend a lot of time in bed, you may not be getting quality sleep. Your body needs both Rapid Eye Movement (REM) sleep and deep sleep. REM sleep, the type during dreaming, helps consolidate memories and is key for learning, creativity, and problem solving. Deep sleep helps repair your body. Both types of sleep can be disrupted during the night, leading to trouble waking and daytime sleepiness.

The problem is, it's hard to know what's really happening while you sleep. You could spend the night in a professional sleep lab hooked up to a bunch of wires and monitors. But a professional sleep study can cost $1,800 without insurance.

A new home sleep monitor called the Zeo Personal Sleep Coach may be a cheaper alternative. This product, which costs from $250 to $350, lets you track your sleep patterns in your own bedroom. You sleep wearing a soft, lightweight headband with sensors that monitor your brain waves and send signals wirelessly to a bedside display. This device, which looks like a clock radio, shows whether you are awake or in light sleep, deep sleep, or REM sleep throughout the night. It also stores that information on a memory card you can upload to a Web site, which helps you review your sleep patterns. You can even get daily coaching tips for better sleep. To find out more about Zeo, go to *www.myzeo.com*.

Surprising cause of dangerous falls

Depression can bring you down — literally. A large Australian study found that seniors with depression and those taking antidepressants were more likely to fall than other older people.

Beware common antidepressants. The researchers looked at more than 20,000 people age 60 and older, comparing those who have taken a tumble to those who haven't. The highest risk of falls was among seniors taking a class of antidepressant drugs called selective serotonin reuptake inhibitors, or SSRIs. Common SSRIs include fluoxetine (Prozac) and sertraline (Zoloft). These seniors had a 50 percent higher risk of falls than others.

Experts say people who are depressed often have an abnormal gait or unusual posture when standing. And it's known that some people on SSRIs experience side effects like dizziness, fatigue, and drowsiness. Even worse, some SSRIs can weaken your bones, making you more prone to fracture if you do fall. But the problem could also be the opposite — dizziness, falls, and possible fractures could contribute to depression.

Watch out for multiple drugs. If you're over age 65 and take four or more drugs regularly, watch your step. You could be two to three times more likely to fall than other seniors, say researchers at the University of North Carolina. They came up with a list of troublemaking drugs that included many prescription antidepressants, seizure drugs, painkillers, and more. The common link is that they all work to depress your central nervous system. That can make you less alert and slower to react.

Even some nonprescription allergy medications, sleep aids, and cold and cough remedies can have similar effects. Basically, anything that can cause drowsiness may put you at risk of falling. So always let your doctor know what over-the-counter medications you're taking, and be sure to read the labels. Ask your doctor about possible alternative remedies. But don't stop taking a prescription drug without talking to your doctor first.

Maintain your balance. More than one-third of seniors fall every year, and two-thirds of those who do get hurt. That's good reason to find out what you can do to lower your risk.

Experts say that if you're depressed, especially if you take antidepressants, you should learn strategies to prevent falls, like balance training and leg-strengthening exercises. You would also benefit from reorganizing your house to reduce hazards, such as adding enough lighting, removing obstacles from walkways, and having railings installed.

Index

for plantar fasciitis 164
for urinary incontinence 251
for wrinkles 311
side effect warning 314
BPH. *See* Benign prostatic
hyperplasia (BPH)
Breakfast, for weight loss 165-171
Breast cancer
aspirin and 249
foods for 231-233
gentle healing for 247
Mediterranean diet to prevent 50
new tests for early detection 250
nutritional supplement warning
241
saturated fat and 233
soy and 234
Brittle bones. *See* Osteoporosis
Broccoli. *See* Sulforaphane
Bronchitis, chronic. *See* Chronic
obstructive pulmonary disease
Brown fat, and weight loss 217
Bunions. *See* Foot pain
Buproprion, for weight loss 229

C

C-reactive protein 55, 68, 74, 76, 77,
110, 147
Caffeine
Alzheimer's disease and 2
energy drinks and 326
exercise and 343
fatigue and 14
kidney stones and 240
monoamine oxidase inhibitors
and 3
Parkinson's disease and 18
Calcium
chocolate warning 124
colon cancer and 196
deficiency and overeating 166
diabetes and 183
guidelines 119
high-protein diet and 167
kidney stones and 240
mineral water and 120
osteoporosis and 118

salt and 119
stroke and 79
supplements 137
Cane, buying and using 152
Capsaicin, for arthritis 152
Carbohydrates
for fatigue 14
for memory 17
for sleep 326
Cardia Salt 63
Cataracts
exercise and 263
free eye exams 275
lutein and zeaxanthin 259
rooibos tea and 255
surgery options 274
ultraviolet (UV) radiation and 264
vitamin C and 79, 256
Cavities. *See also* Dental health
beverages that prevent 277
xylitol and 281
Celiac disease and joint pain 132
Cereal
for depression 14
for weight loss 167
heart disease and stroke 80
Charoset, health benefits 65
Chemical peel 311
Cherries
for arthritis 128
for muscle loss 319
for sleep 325
for weight loss 180
Chia, health benefits 89
Chili peppers, for weight loss 173
Chiropractic therapy
for chronic pain 335
for high blood pressure 97
Chlorinated water, and bladder
cancer 247
Chocolate
arthritis and 132
bone density and 124
for weight loss 172
health benefits 54
Chocolate milk, for muscle loss 319
Choline, health benefits 232

Chondroitin, for arthritis 135
Chronic obstructive pulmonary
    disease (COPD)
    help for symptoms 354
    inhaled medications warning 362
    nutritional tips 327-329
Chronic pain
    alternative therapies 335-337
    drug side effects 356-358
    electrical stimulation for 360-362
    exercise for 339
    herbs for 332-334
    omega-3 fatty acids for 331
    prolotherapy for 358-360
    social support for 339
    vitamin D for 317
Cinnamon, for high blood pressure
    62, 66
Clostridium difficile (C. difficile) 113
Coenzyme Q10
    for tinnitus 261
    for weight loss 200
Coffee
    caution 59
    cavities and 277
    diabetes and 197, 198
    exercise and 343
    for gallstones 198
    gout and 126
    heart disease warning 57
    kidney stones and 240
    osteoporosis and 126
    Parkinson's disease and 18
    stress and 14
    stroke and 59, 79
Cold medicines, caution 98
Collagen injections
    for urinary incontinence 251
    for wrinkles 313
Colon cancer
    aspirin for 230
    dairy for 196
    exercise for 211
    fruits, veggies, and legumes for 190
    high insulin levels and 190
    krill oil for 87
    omega-3 fatty acids for 187

screening tests 224
    turmeric for 194
Compact fluorescent bulbs (CFLs),
    and skin problems 300
Congestive heart failure
    hawthorn for 89
    hip fracture risk and 162
    omega-3 fatty acids and 52
Conjugated linoleic acid, for weight
    loss 199
Continuous Positive Airway
    Pressure (CPAP), for sleep apnea
    220
CoQ10. *See* Coenzyme Q10
Cornmeal, for smoother skin 298
Corns and calluses. *See* Foot pain
Coronary bypass surgery 111
Cranberry
    for dental health 279
    to prevent cancer 238
Cruciferous vegetables, health
    benefits 76, 232, 238
Curcumin. *See* Turmeric

D

Dairy food
    diabetes and 182-184
    for colon cancer 196
    for weight loss 167
    kidney stones and 240
Deep vein thrombosis (DVT),
    HEPA filter for 101
Dehydration
    dizziness and 323
    wrinkles and 291
Dementia. *See* Alzheimer's disease
Dental health. *See also* Cavities
    enamel-eroding foods 279-281
    mouthwash warning 283
    teeth whitening 285
    toothbrush care 282, 284
    X-ray caution 284
Denture cream, and zinc overdose 347
Depression
    antidepressant caution 365
    antioxidant vitamins for 15
    bright light for 40

Fatigue *(continued)*
  breakfast and 14
  exercise for 211
  quercetin for 324
Fem-Dophilus, for yeast infections 242
Fiber
  age-related macular degeneration
    and 257
  lung function and 328
  weight loss and 179
Fibromyalgia
  exercise for 340
  prolotherapy for 358
Fish. *See* Omega-3 fatty acids
Fish oil supplements 6, 88, 331. *See
  also* Omega-3 fatty acids
Flat feet. *See* Foot pain
Flaxseed
  health benefits 72
  omega-3 fatty acids and 53
Flaxseed oil
  heart attack and stroke risk 72
  prostate cancer warning 235
  wrinkles and 294
Folate
  health benefits 9
  sources of 10
Folic acid supplements. *See also* Folate
  age-related macular degeneration
    and 261
  hearing loss and 260
  stroke and 85
Foot pain 154
Fosamax (alendronate) warning 127,
  160
French paradox 56

G

Gallbladder disease, hormone
  therapy and 228
Gallstones, coffee for 198
Garlic
  for Alzheimer's disease 8
  for benign prostatic hyperplasia
    (BPH) 238
  for heart disease 48
  for high cholesterol 62

Gastritis, sulforaphane for 192
Genistein supplement, cancer warning 241
Ginger, for high cholesterol 62
Ginkgo
  for stroke 89
  memory and 19
Ginseng
  for diabetes 202-204
  for impotence 245
Glaucoma
  exercise and 264
  new screening test 273
Glucosamine
  for arthritis 135
  for wrinkles 295
Glycemic index 187-190
Goldenroot, for depression 25
Gotu kola, for Alzheimer's disease 21
Gout
  coffee and 126
  high-fructose corn syrup 134
  vitamin C for 127
Grape juice, for Alzheimer's disease 4
Grapes
  for weight loss 181
  health benefits 56
  memory and 4
Green tea
  Alzheimer's disease and 2
  cavities and 277
  for Sjogren's syndrome 278
  for weight loss 61, 172
  gum disease and 277
  high blood pressure and 60
  osteoporosis and 118
  Parkinson's disease and 2
  skin cancer and 288
  stroke and 79
  wrinkles and 287
Gum
  colorectal surgery and 225
  to control cravings 210
Gum-grafting surgery 286

H

H. pylori, and digestive problems 193

Hair loss
  aromatherapy oils for 309
  iron for 65
Hammertoes. *See* Foot pain
Harmonica, for easier breathing 354
Hawthorn, health benefits 89
Head and neck cancers, preventing 281
Headaches
  prolotherapy for 358
  stroke and 103, 105
  TMJ and 266
Hearing aids, buying 269
Hearing loss
  buying a hearing aid 269
  cell phone radiation and 266
  drug side effects and 268
  loud noise and 265
  stroke and 102
  supplements for 260
Heart attack
  automated external defibrillator (AED) for 106
  broccoli and 76
  coffee to prevent 59
  egg caution 169
  omega-3 fatty acids and 52
  pneumonia vaccine and 114
  Prilosec warning 111
  red yeast rice and 90
  tomatoes and 75
  vitamin D to prevent 70
  warning signs 104
Heart disease
  acrylamides and 68
  angioplasty vs. coronary bypass surgery 111
  B-vitamin supplements and 85
  breakfast benefits 57
  coffee warning 57
  dark chocolate for 54
  garlic for 48
  HEPA filter for 101
  high-fructose corn syrup and 177
  krill oil for 87
  leafy greens for 70

  low-dose aspirin therapy for 108
  low-fat milk and 70
  Mediterranean diet and 47
  nuts for 51
  omega-3 fatty acids for 52
  plastic containers and 107
  Polymeal and 47
  quercetin and 56
  resveratrol for 55, 56
  saturated fats 54
  sea vegetables and 77
  sweetened beverages and 74
  tomatoes for 74
  trans fats and 54
  whole grains and 58, 71, 80
Heart failure. *See* Congestive heart failure
Heart surgery caution 111-113
Heartburn
  melatonin for 206
  Prilosec warning 111, 204
Heel pain. *See* Plantar fasciitis
Hemochromatosis 161
HEPA filter, health benefits 101
Herbal supplements
  for arthritis 143-145
  for heart health 89
  for memory loss 20
Herbal tea, for high blood pressure 61
Herpes simplex virus type 1, and Alzheimer's disease 44
High blood pressure
  Alzheimer's disease and 33
  chiropractic therapy for 97
  coffee warning 60
  cold medicines and 98
  dark chocolate for 54
  dizziness and 347
  green tea for 60
  herbal tea with hibiscus for 61
  herbs and spices for 62
  low-dose aspirin therapy for 108
  low-fat milk for 70
  lupin kernel flour for 73
  massage for 97
  Mediterranean diet and 49

Laparoscopic adjustable gastric banding, for weight loss 226
Laser skin resurfacing 311
Laughter, for stress 100
Leafy greens, health benefits 76
Legumes, for colon cancer 190
Lemon juice, for age spots 298
Linoleic acid 51, 291. *See also* Omega-6 fatty acids
Linolenic acid 72. *See also* Omega-3 fatty acids
Lupin kernel flour, health benefits 73
Lycopene
  apricots and 64
  emphysema and 328
  for prostate cancer 237
  skin cancer and 292
  tomatoes and 75, 117

M

Magnesium 121
  colon cancer and 196
  diabetes and 182
  for hearing loss 261
  for sleep 326
  osteoporosis and 121
Massage
  for chronic pain 336
  for high blood pressure 97
MC-FAQ screening test for Alzheimer's disease 42
Mediterranean diet
  Alzheimer's disease and 49
  Alzheimer's disease and 8
  heart disease and 47
Melatonin
  for heartburn 206
  for sleep 325
Memory loss. *See also* Alzheimer's disease
  anticholinergic drugs and 45
  B vitamins and 10
  calorie restriction for 13
  carbohydrates and 17
  ginkgo and 19
  herbal supplements for 20
  Juvenon for 22

  sleep and 38
  soy and 16
Memory, improving 34, 36, 38, 342
Mental decline. *See* Alzheimer's disease
Menthol, for arthritis 152
Mercury, in seafood 51
Metabolic syndrome
  exercise and 209
  kidney stones and 249
  low-fat milk for 70
  nuts for 50
Methicillin-resistant *Staphylococcus aureus* (MRSA) 113, 305
Methylmalonic acid, and mental decline 10
Microdermabrasion 312
Migraines. *See* Headaches
Mineral water, calcium and 120
Monocolin A 90
Monounsaturated fats
  bone density and 117
  for heart health 297
  sources of 50
  stop cravings 186
Monterey Sun-Bella mushrooms 71
Morton Lite Salt 63
MSG (monosodium glutamate) and obesity 173
Mudpacks, for arthritis 151
Multivitamin supplements, pros and cons 81, 243
Muscle loss
  foods to prevent 319-321
  protein powders for 321
  supplements for 329
  weight lifting for 340
Music, health benefits 41, 95

N

Natto. *See* Soy
Natural sugars, for diabetes 192
NeuroStar, for depression 46
Niacin. *See* Vitamin B3
Niacor 85
Niaspan 85
Nicotinamide. *See* Vitamin B3

NightWave Sleep Assistant 353
Nintendo Wii. *See* Video games, for brain health
NSAID creams, for arthritis 152
Nuts
  breast cancer and 232
  for diabetes 184
  health benefits 50

O

Oatmeal
  for dry skin 297
  for lower cholesterol 58
  for weight loss 166
Oleic acid, and appetite 186
Olive oil. *See also* Monounsaturated fats; Omega-3 fatty acids
  breast cancer and 232
  cooking tip 53
  for arthritis 132
  for bone density 117
  for heart disease 47
  for high blood pressure 49
  for skin moisturizing 297
Omega-3 fatty acids
  age-related macular degeneration and 257
  Alzheimer's disease and 5, 79
  arrhythmias and 53
  as a brain booster 5
  colon cancer and 187
  depression and 5
  dry eyes and 258
  for arthritis 129-131
  for chronic pain 331
  for diabetes 186
  for heart health 52
  for kidney stones 239
  krill oil 87
  Parkinson's disease and 5
  prostate cancer and 234
  sea vegetables and 77
  seafood caution 51
  skin cancer and 293
  sources of 6, 53, 66
  wrinkles and 294

Omega-6 fatty acids
  Alzheimer's disease and 7
Oolong tea
  as a brain booster 2
  cavities and 277
Oral cancer
  coffee and 278
  mouthwash warning 283
Orlistat (Alli), for weight loss 229
Osteoarthritis. *See* Arthritis
Osteomalacia, causes 139
Osteonecrosis of the jaw 160
Osteopenia, drug guidelines 159
Osteoporosis
  alendronate (Fosamax) warning 127, 160
  alkaline supplement for 116
  calcium for 118
  coffee and 126
  congestive heart failure and 162
  fruits and veggies for 116
  green tea for 60
  L-carnitine for 141
  low-dose aspirin for 161
  magnesium for 121
  mineral water for 120
  monounsaturated fats for 117
  osteopenia drug guidelines 159
  potassium and 119
  resveratrol and 123
  salt and 119
  silicon and 126
  soy and 124
  tea for 118
  vitamin C for 128
Osteotomy, for arthritis 158
Overactive bladder. *See* Urinary incontinence

P

Pain. *See* Chronic pain
Parkinson's disease
  anticholinergic drugs warning 45
  coffee for 18
  fish to prevent 4
  green tea and 2, 61
  iron and 17

statins for 44
vitamin D and 12
vitamin E for 18
Percutaneous coronary intervention.
See Angioplasty
Percutaneous ultrasound guided
approach, for plantar fasciitis 163
Periodontitis, yogurt for 278
Peripheral arterial disease (PAD),
walking and 100
Phosphorus supplements, for kid-
ney stones 242
Physical activity. *See* Exercise
Pillar palatal implants, for sleep
apnea 221
Plantar fasciitis 154, 163
Plastic containers, heart disease and
107
Plavix (clopidogrel) caution 111
Pneumonia vaccine, heart attack
and 114
Polychlorinated biphenyls (PCBs),
in seafood 51
Polymeal, to prevent heart disease 47
Pomegranate juice
for arthritis 133
for dental health 279
for prostate cancer 237
Potassium
apricots and 64
bananas and 65
osteoporosis and 119
salt substitutes and 63
Prayer, long-term care and 28
Prilosec (omeprazole) caution 111
Probiotic pill, for yeast infections 242
Prolotherapy 358-360
Prostate cancer
lycopene for 237
obesity and 248
omega-3 fatty acids for 234
PSA (prostate specific antigen)
blood test 253
sulforaphane for 238
vitamin E warning 243
PSA. *See* Prostate cancer

Psoriasis
health problems and 307
honey for 297
stress and 301
supplement for 296
turmeric for 195
Pterostilbene, health benefits 4, 56
Pycnogenol
diabetes and 202
for arthritis 144

Q

Quercetin
for fatigue 324
health benefits 56

R

Radar breast imaging 251
Restless legs syndrome
diphenhydramine caution 358
exercise for 353
iron deficiency and 334
valerian for 332
Resveratrol
bone density and 123
for breast cancer 231
for weight loss 201
heart disease and 55, 56
skin cancer and 293
Resvinatrol Complete 57, 201
Retinol, for wrinkles 304
Rheumatoid arthritis. *See* Arthritis
Rooibos tea, for diabetic cataracts
and retinopathy 255
Rose hips, for arthritis 144
Roux-en-Y gastric bypass, for
weight loss 226

S

S-adenosylmethionine. *See* SAM-e
Saffron, for depression 9
Sage, for Alzheimer's disease 8
Salicylate, for arthritis 152
Salt
guidelines 63
kidney stones and 240
osteoporosis and 119

Sunshine vitamin. *See* Vitamin D

Superbugs 113, 289, 305

Surgery caution 113

T

Tai chi, health benefits 94, 148, 247, 308, 349

Tea. *See* Black tea; Green tea; Oolong tea; Rooibos tea

Teeth. *See* Dental health; Cavities

Tempe. *See* Soy

Temporomandibular joint (TMJ) disorders, and tinnitus 266

Tesofensine, for weight loss 228

Theanine, as a brain booster 2

Tinnitus
    Coenzyme Q10 for 261
    treatments for 266-268, 270

Tofu. *See* Soy

Trans fats, types of 54

Trans vaccenic acids 54

Transcranial magnetic stimulation
    for depression 46
    for tinnitus 271

Transcutaneous electrical nerve stimulation (TENS) 360

Turmeric
    diabetic retinopathy and 256
    for Alzheimer's disease 8
    for heart disease 63
    health benefits 193-196

TYM screening test for Alzheimer's disease 43

Type 2 diabetes. *See* Diabetes

U

Ulcers
    curcumin supplements for 195
    sulforaphane for 193

Ultraviolet (UV) radiation
    and vision problems 264
    compact fluorescent bulbs (CFLs) and 300
    skin cancer and 293
    wrinkles and 287, 294, 302

Unicompartmental knee arthroplasty, for arthritis 158

Uric acid 18

Urinary incontinence
    anticholinergic drugs warning 45, 252
    foods to avoid 236
    injections for 251
    self-help 246

V

Valerian
    for anxiety 25
    for restless legs syndrome 332

Vanilla extract, warning 66

Varicose veins 99

Vascular dementia, high blood pressure and 33

Vegetarian eating plan 69

Venous thrombosis, migraines and 103

Ventricular tachycardia. *See* Arrhythmia

Video games, for brain health 37

Vitamin B12
    Alzheimer's disease and 10
    depression and 11, 15
    osteoporosis and 121
    Prilosec warning 204

Vitamin B3
    Alzheimer's disease and 11
    high cholesterol and 84
    skin cancer and 293
    supplement warning 86

Vitamin C
    bone density and 128
    cancer warning 241
    cataracts and 79, 256
    for arthritis 127
    for depression 15
    for gout 127
    for stroke 58
    wrinkles and 290

Vitamin D
    age-related macular degeneration and 258
    Alzheimer's disease and 12
    colon cancer and 197
    depression and 12